EAT TO BE FREE!

E.A. ORDOÑEZ, M.D.

with Alexandra J. Zani

Eat to Be Free!

Published in the United States of America.

ISBN: 978-1-257-02289-2

Edited by M.F.A. Shipp

Eat to Be Free!

Table of Contents

DEDICATION

This book is dedicated to all my patients who successfully participated in my lifestyle change/weight management plan during the past twenty years. It is dedicated to those who have stepped out of the box of traditional methods of weight loss and made a commitment to the lifestyle changes that I recommended to finally improve their health and quality of longevity. It is through this commitment that they saw the possibility of experiencing a slimmer, healthier, and happier outcome. It is through the recommendation and repeated requests of my patients that I write this book.

There were individuals along my journey of life who contributed to my personal growth, development and success throughout the years. My parents supported me during my earlier education at the medical school in Manila and encouraged me to venture across the Pacific Ocean to come to the United States to pursue my medical career. I especially want to thank my father, Alfred L. Ordoñez, who said, "Just study, son."

My practice administrator, Edisa Sukurica, has been a considerable asset in the daily success of my office. Her meticulous attention to details has been invaluable to me and my patients.

And especially to Alexandra Zani, my valuable consultant in researching the data for this text, who also guided the rewriting and making of this book.

Through the unconditional love and support of my whole family, this book has become a reality that I am able to share with patients, colleagues and new readers.

Ernie A. Ordonez, M.D.

August 2010

PREFACE

There is a pressing need for personal change centered around a common theme of individual fulfillment and wholeness. By extension, there is a requirement for wellness and balance in an age of extremism and/or self focus that should inspire us to become engaged in personal learning about health improvement and maintenance. The rising obesity rates herald an increase in the resultant health problems, such as diabetes, metabolic syndrome, hypertension and its complications, all of which are interconnected with mental health concerns. Compounding these are the troubling statistics associated with overweight adolescents, teens, and young adults with burgeoning obesity and the associated rise in mood disorders, etc. The resultant loss of community, collective support and empathy has produced isolation and self-introspection, without a sense of connectedness to the common good, which creates a setting for poverty of purpose and focus.

How do we regain our footing, our reach for healthy living and behaviors? It begins with changing our attitudes, improving our health perspectives and increasing our self-efficacy as we encourage those around us to join into the celebration of better living and investment in life. The purpose of this book is to begin the journey back to overall wellness through improving our physical health from the inside out. It provides food for thought that reaches far beyond the words on each page. We must not just learn information, but, personalize and activate what we read and hear. Indeed optimal health resides within the heart and mind of each individual.

Kim Bullock, M.D.

Director of Fellowships, Director of Community Health Division, Assistant Director of Service-Learning, Associate Clinical Professor, Department of Family Medicine
Georgetown Medical Center, Washington, D.C.

INTRODUCTION

During the past two decades, I have devoted myself to focusing on this very important disease plaguing the 21st Century -- OBESITY. In 1984, the U.S. obesity rate was less than 20% (CDC, 2010).[1] Current studies indicate that more than two thirds of U.S. adults -190 million Americans- are overweight, one third of which are considered obese, with more than 10% of being children and adolescents. These numbers continue to rise.[2] A new 2007-2008 report showed that a combined male and female obesity and overweight statistics was 68%, with more women than men, 35.5% vs. 32.2%. A January 2010 report now shows that men now at 72.3% with women at 64.1%.[3] More staggering is the 140 billion dollar price tag burdening our current health care system.[4]

Since 1975, and prior to my focus on weight loss as a national and personal concern, I followed the traditional methods of disease management that were taught during my medical school and residency training along with the recommendations presented through the hospital systems and medical associations. And, in particular, there were no seminars and/or programs on nutrition, prevention and weight loss.

While working as a general practitioner during the 1980s, I discovered that the majority of patient ailments became more complicated, instead of experiencing improvements and greater well-being. They were walking the rocky path of at-risk Lifestyle habits, increased levels of stress, poor eating habits and sedentary Lifestyle leading to increased weight gain and obesity.

The message became clearer during my early mornings of making the patient rounds in the hospital. Instead of getting well, so many patients plummeted into having more physical complications, which in turn forced increased medications and even additional surgery. This also meant waiting for various approval levels and scrutiny from insurance companies and other hierarchal echelons within the system. A patient's immune system became so compromised beyond what his/her body could tolerate, that an early death was inevitable. Excessive weight placed an undue burden on a patient's ability to work, positioning even more responsibility on their families and the healthcare system locally with mounting costs.

I began to notice a common denominator among my patients. Whenever their weight increased by 10 to 15 pounds above their ideal size, (above a BMI of 25) they began to experience increased health risks — higher blood pressure, elevated sugar levels, indigestion, inflammation, hormone imbalances, reduced immune system with an inability to handle stress leading to further hormonal and emotional interruptions.

Radical changes began to happen in the early 1980s with the HMO, PPO and other insurance companies who began to place higher controls onto the medical field. At the same time women patients began to ask me to assist them to lose weight. I knew very little about it except to give them diet sheets to follow. Insurance companies denied claims for the overweight. Yet the correlation between weight gain and chronic ailments was becoming progressively more evident and now in 2010 it is fully understood.

It was also during this time that newly organized movements began to manifest through the efforts of several insightful physicians and other healthcare professionals. They realized that our traditional health care system was killing people. In 1996, I joined the American Academy of Anti-Aging Medicine (A4M), a worldwide organization of physicians and health professional with more than 20,000 members. The A4M became a world bank of scientific research and studies, and continues to introduce new scientific data and research for longevity and prevention of debilitating diseases. The A4M believes that *"the disabilities associated with normal aging are caused by physiological dysfunction which in many cases is ameliorable to medical treatment, such that the human lifespan can be increased, and the quality of one's life enhanced as one grows chronologically older."*

Personally, I was no longer willing to continue in a system that did not place focus on PREVENTION and in one that denied the fact that weight loss was a major health threat that required medical care as a new American disease. Most of the ailments that I treated with my patients during my earlier practice were totally preventable. This was unequivocally summarized by former Surgeon General, (2002-2006) Richard Carmona, M.D. and Chairperson of Partnership to Fight Chronic Disease. During his term as Surgeon General, Dr. Carmona made a statement that we must have healthy Americans by 2010; that isn't happening yet. As part of the 2009 administration, he commented:

"Our current healthcare system is a 'sick care' system with perverse incentives." The disease and economic burden that we have upon us – we currently spend more than $2 trillion per year on health care, or 16% of our gross domestic product – is largely preventable .... We need a paradigm shift that moves our nation to one that embraces health and wellness through appropriated prevention strategies and builds an infrastructure that begins to reward health care providers who want to keep our citizens healthy."

Throughout the past 20 years of my weight management practice, what I learned from the experts in the field has enabled me to gain great insight and an understanding of the entire aging process as well as the devastation on health and quality of living due to obesity and poor lifestyle habits. This education helped me to become more dedicated and grow a deep commitment that allows me to assist my patients to lose weight effectively, safely and successfully.

When I decided to embark on my studies in the field of weight loss, a series of questions came to mind:

1. What is my role as a physician?
2. How can I persuade my over weight/obese patients to understand the risks?
3. How do I counsel and encourage my patients to become committed to do something that they know they can do,

but have made excuses to avoid doing, despite knowing the benefits?

I realized that I had to integrate and expand a new way of thinking — a new personal paradigm shift — into an expanded thought process beyond what I learned as a physician. I attended many leadership seminars, listened to numerous motivational speakers, attended medical conventions, and read emerging books and journals on the topic. I examined my own role in converting a general medical practice into one of weight loss with focused strategies and maintenance programs. I called it a "lifestyle health plan". It is through these endeavors that I discovered a profound truth about having a very successful weight loss practice.

Indeed, in the latter part of the '80s, I was able to manage my parents' medical conditions. I brought both of them from the Philippines to Jacksonville, Florida, in order to oversee their treatment. My father, who was Type I diabetic, had hypertensive heart disease and osteoarthritis in his knees; my mother also had hypertensive heart disease. Both were obese. Their improvements due to my weight loss program and supervision were incredibly pronounced: Both were free from illness and the drugs needed for management.

To the readers who are evaluating these words, I invite you to scan the media on this topic of dieting. Read the books, tabloids, magazines, listen to radio interviews and watch TV programs. You may notice conflicting theories or outwardly quick remedies. However, in order for you to lose weight you have to recognize that there is a great connection between how you think and how you live the rest of your life. Be mindful that ***Eat to Be Free!*** is a complete and efficient guide, particularly in addressing the way that you think and speak. I invite you to examine the "WHY" and follow the program in every detail to effectively experience a permanent body makeover. You must transform the mind first so that your reason for losing the weight becomes a permanent Lifestyle change. You are the only person who can influence how your life will emerge in order to successfully maintain the only item that is most valuable to you — YOUR HEALTH.

You are also the only one who can enjoy the good life and pursue your own happiness.

I hope and trust that you will go on until the priceless blessing of perfect health is yours for a lifetime.

Faithfully yours forever,

Ernesto A. Ordonez, M.D.

August 2010

MY TRANSFORMATION: THE CHALLENGE

The transition from traditional or conventional medicine to what I now call functional medicine was not a comfortable decision. After practicing family medicine and general surgery for years, I decided to pursue a weight management practice.

Creating a weight loss program was challenging, but my decision to do that very thing grew from repeated requests by my patients to have a weight loss regimen designed for them. Their needs led me to create and develop a purpose-driven system and a program consisting of food and exercise plans. Both the system and the program are discussed in my strategy, which I outline in the following chapters.

During my initial research for the system, I discovered the use of "diet pills" or appetite suppressant drugs that were approved by the Food and Drug Administration (FDA). I knew little about any of these, as I had never prescribed any during my original practice. However, since I was licensed to prescribe drugs for diabetes, hypertension, arthritis, depression, insomnia, birth control pills, and medications for cardiac and other conditions, I knew I was able to prescribe diet pills as well. So, I decided to implement such drugs in my program to make it much easier for patients to follow the food plan.

Profiling a drug or drugs to be used in the system was a task as well. Appetite suppressant drugs must be safe and effective, with few side effects, or none at all. With the assistance of a friend, a librarian of a local hospital (where I was a member of the medical staff) provided upon request all the information I needed on most diet pills on the market. I chose Ionamin® and Pondimin® from among these for testing.[5]

I tested these drugs first on myself, taking 15 milligrams (mg.) of Ionamin® (Phentermine) in the morning after breakfast and 20 milligrams of Pondimin® (Fenfluramine) at night before dinner. I experienced very minimal side-effects and found I tolerated both drugs quite well; I simply needed to drink plenty of water and eat more fruit. After two weeks of this regimen, I lost 10 pounds or more. I then called some of my patients who had requested the weight loss program, to see if they were interested in having these drugs prescribed for them.

By the late 1980s, I decided to devote my entire practice to weight loss management.

By 1992, as reported by Dr. Michael Weintraub, these two drugs had become familiar and effective drugs for weight loss, popularly known as "Phen-Fen". Indeed, they were the best combination of diet drugs. Here in the U.S. and around the world, Phen-Fen was a sensation, a household word. The fate of Phen-Fen was to be a sudden end, however. On September 15, 1997, the FDA banned use of Fenfluramine (Pondimin®) and its sister drug Redux, but has permitted the use of Phentermine until the present.

Just to share a personal note here with my readers and some of my patients who remember this event in my practice, between 1989 and 1992, I was under investigation by the Drug Enforcement Administration (DEA) and the Board of Medicine about this combined usage of the two drugs. Nothing came of this investigation, since no patients under my care in my weight loss program were injured or experienced any side effects or adverse reactions.

Most, if not all, patients stopped coming to my office after the news came out about reported adverse reactions to the heart and lungs due to Pondimin® (Fenfluramine). My office load dropped to a few patients a day. My office staff was cut from six to just one — my daughter Cristina.

I was not discouraged at all, since it was my determination to be an expert in weight loss management. It was my vision that someday I would create a mission to have a community of healthy people through my weight loss management.

Today, word of mouth brings patients (we prefer to call them guests) to my office to seek assistance. I know without a doubt, that experience is, indeed, the best education in life.

This is functional medicine. To it, and to you, I am committed.

I

ORDOÑEZ' STRATEGIES FOR WEIGHT LOSS

"Nothing tastes as good as thin feels"

ଓଃ

ONE ✧ THE ROLE OF THE PHYSICIAN IN WEIGHT LOSS

"The doctor of the future will give no medicine, but will interest her or his patients in the care of the human frame, in proper diet, and in the cause and prevention of disease."

Thomas A. Edison
U.S. Inventor (1847-1931)

The issue of obesity is challenging to both the patient and her or his physician. A patient may end up at the doctor's office for an urgent health concern that tends to take precedence over its actual underlying cause — obesity. Given the time constraints of most doctors, including the cost of malpractice, the pressing health concern usually ends up taking precedence during a consultation. Overweight and obesity may not be part of the discussion.

The February 2009 issue of *Medical Economics* points out that many physicians are hesitant to discuss weight management with their patients. Obesity isn't always recorded on charts, as evidenced that only one in five obese patients are actually documented. When it is diagnosed, however, patients were more than likely to development a weight management program with their doctor.

Years ago while I was working weekends in a local emergency room, the majority of patients being admitted were obese with concerns of high blood pressure, diabetes, back pain, and high cholesterol. It was obvious that their real issue was excessive weight. I encouraged them to come to my office so that I could properly assist them.

Additionally, during their examination in the ER, it quickly became apparent that all they wanted were refills for their medication even when I reviewed their risks of heart attack, stroke, and heart failure. Weekend after weekend this scenario continued with one or two patients having a fatal heart attack.

Few patients said their doctors discussed their weight problems. The concern was more about their immediate affliction, thus prescribing medication to get it under control. The underlying cause was not discussed.

It did not take long for the hospital administrator to come to me and told me to stop telling patients in the ER to lose weight. I found myself facing the hospital staff regarding this issue. I resigned.

Scope of Concern

Despite the fact that obesity translates into a higher risk factor for debilitating diseases, it is not discussed — WHY?

One reason is that a person's weight can be a sensitive topic. The patient may take offense if the topic is discussed.

Further talk may open a door for more discussion or other concerns, including possible treatment strategies such as bariatric surgery or other measures, all of which may pose a higher liability.

The scope of concern expands if preventative measures are not taken with at-risk patients. Primary care doctors could experience even greater liability issues if a patient is likely diagnosed with a disease for which obesity is a risk factor OR when they resort to a high-risk option of bariatric medicine. If a patient reaches the point of bariatric surgery, the issue becomes extreme, with increased liability and possible death.

What if the patient suffers a heart attack? Was it preventable through an initial diagnosis of the potential risk factor (obesity)?

Encouraging discussion during the consultation can lead to preventing catastrophic consequences later. It is one more good reason to work with at risk patients BEFORE their diseases burden an already overfull health care system.

Obesity and Stigmatization

There are well researched and documented studies confirming that obese individuals experience higher rates of depression, anxiety, social isolation, and poorer psychological adjustment. Some overweight individuals may internalize and accept the negative attitudes developed from their own personal thoughts as well as from other critical individuals. This continues to lower personal self esteem and the ability to feel comfortable and get along in society. They may respond by eating more food and continue in a lifestyle that perpetuates their dilemma.

Overweight/obese individuals can also be shunned from employment due to potential health liability and perceived lowering of company image.

Health professionals can help reduce these stigmas by working with their overweight and obese adult and child patients. There are some specific guidelines pointed out by *The Obesity Society*, an organization whose focus provides support to health practitioners. These guidelines, as well as my own, become an integral component of my training program when educating physicians who are contemplating adding in a weight loss program to their practice. Prior to taking on this responsibility, it is important to examine one's own attitudes and biases towards the obese.

1. Do I make assumptions based on weight regarding a person's character, intelligence, professional success, health status, or lifestyle behaviors?

2. Am I comfortable working with people of all shapes and size?
3. Am I sensitive to the needs and concerns of obese individuals?
4. Do I treat the individual or only the condition? Is prevention part of my program and do I "practice what I preach"?

TWO ℘ PROGRAM PROFILE - WEIGHT LOSS

When contemplating a plan for weight loss, a key component for you to consider is to examine several factors surrounding your investment. The success of your program is highly reliant on partnering with a physician who has the expertise, dedication, and passion for operating a weight loss program.

1. The plan must effectively address your medical problem(s), including weight.
2. Focus should just not be on what is read on the scale. A program should have the ability of dealing with the psychological issues, including the underlying <u>causes</u> that contribute to your weight condition.
3. Does it take into account your previous weight loss history and identify the effectiveness of, and your response to, those programs.
4. What was your experience? Was there a positive and supportive environment?
5. Was the health care professional sensitive to your history? Did s/he customize a program to meet your needs?
6. Did you comply with his/her directives or blame him/her if you experienced poor success?
7. Realistic goals should be determined. Patients become excited when they participate in a program that begins to work in their favor from the beginning.

8. The physician and his/her staff should be supportive at all times. A weight loss environment requires confidentiality and respect for each patient.
9. When there is a large amount of weight loss to consider, an individual requires professional help to monitor the changes that occur during this period.
10. COST: The total investment of the program should be conveyed in the first visit including outlining the cost for return visits (weekly or bi-monthly).
11. Discuss any dietary prescription medication such as appetite suppressants. Instructions and any side effects must be outlined.
12. The program should provide authoritative information about the food plan including nutrition, exercise and the benefits of the entire plan.
13. There must be a strong support and maintenance component. This requires reinforcement and motivation.

A Paradigm Shift – The System

Know Your WHYS: Your reasons, intentions and desires propel you or drive you to do this program. They have to be important enough.

Attitude: Change. Did the health care practitioner acknowledge the difficulty of lifestyle changes and convey that? Your attitude can take you to new heights. It can make you or break you. Take a chance, for it will make you grow and become a better you.

Belief: Believe in yourself. Do things that you believe are worth doing, as long as you know that the outcome is beneficial to yourself.

Commitment: Have a strong desire to endure the pains and small sacrifices in order to reap the health benefits over time.

THREE ᘓ GUIDELINES FOR HEALTHY EATING

> *"Eat breakfast like a king, like a queen for lunch and like a pauper for supper"*
>
> German Proverb

My food plan is simple: This is not a D-I-E-(T).

Part of a good weight loss program is to come to the realization that you should develop lifestyle changes and eating habits that support you both emotionally, physically and mentally. Food is the fuel of the brain and the body. It's not about going "on and off" a diet; it's about transforming your attitude towards food and Lifestyle. A key component is to plan out when you are going to eat and then make the correct food choices. Going to extremes in food plans — specialized food, packaged frozen foods and artificial drinks — does not always support a positive outcome.

1. Eat a large breakfast with the focus on carbohydrates. This is fuel for the brain and creates energy. This is the most important meal of the day. You will feel better and have more energy throughout the day. Eat your fruits before your breakfast.

2. Eat your main meal around 1:30-2:00 in the afternoon; be sure that it incorporates protein and other nutritional food, particularly vegetables.

3. Supper should be consumed before 6:00 when possible, and should consist of small amounts of protein and vegetables. Never go to bed digesting protein or a heavy meal, as it places undue stress on your body.

4. Snacks can consist of fruits, raw vegetables, and nuts such as almonds, peanuts and mixed nuts.

5. Beverages: Drink fresh pure water — eight-ten 8-oz. glasses — every day, and keep yourself well hydrated. Avoid soft drinks, diet drinks, energy drinks, artificially sweetened and/or colored drinks, and too much caffeine. Also, be sure to include fruits that are juicy, as their naturally organized water, sugars, fiber, vitamins and enzymes help preserve your youthful appearance.

"Water is the only drink for a wise man — it is the elixir of Life."— Henry David Thoreau

In my opinion, when you are healthy, you become recession-resistant, and of course, disease-resistant.

FOUR ☙ EXERCISE, EXERCISE, EXERCISE

Exercise is essential to the preservation of health. Inactivity is a strong cause of physical wasting and degeneration. The vigor and quality of maintaining good circulation supports the aeration of the blood, brings nutrients to every organ of the body, including good muscular activity.

Spend ten to fifteen minutes on a treadmill, or thirty minutes of brisk walking. Do this every day, ideally between the hours of 5:30 – 10:00 every morning, since the metabolism continues to rise throughout the day. Exercise consisting of any activity, including physical work, helps provide mental alertness as well as energy for the entire day.

I highly recommend a treadmill as a simple, structured exercise in my program. Just ten minutes every morning contributes to your maintaining optimum energy levels throughout the day. People naturally quit exercising because they are doing it for too long and become bored. Taking ten minutes out of twenty four hours is more appealing and achievable.

Excessive and overzealous exercise is not recommended since it may have adverse effects on your muscles. It's the consistency of exercise – even for small time duration — that makes the difference.

Exercise is the best antidote to aging. It keeps you alert and enhances your reaction time. It prevents dementia. It stimulates your immune system. It energizes your cardiovascular system, and improves the sensitivity of target tissue to insulin and thyroid hormones. It prevents cardiovascular disease. It reduces blood pressure. It improves the quality of sleep, and helps alleviate depression. Exercise helps retard bone loss and reduces risk of osteoporosis.

Additionally, exercise improves cerebral circulation, enhances sexual performance, and improves self-esteem. Imagine getting these benefits with just fifteen minutes a day! WOW — you will feel great!

FIVE ☙ APPETITE SUPPRESSANTS

Obesity/overweight is truly a compulsive behavioral disorder contracted by an act of will. I have found that this disorder can be managed by combining pharmacological agents such as appetite suppressant medication, along with a life-style change food program.

My experience as a physician is that the use of an appetite suppressant is a must in order to assist patients in easing their transition from one lifestyle to another in their quest to lose weight effectively, safely and successfully. Profiling patients during the initiation of the program assists me in the use of a specific appetite suppressant medication.

It is important that time is spent with patients in explaining the modes of actions of the medications and any possible side effects. I emphasize my availability to them for any issue that might be of concern or for any drug reactions. Knowing they can reach me anytime is indeed a reassuring factor to patients.

SIX ☙ FOLLOW-UP AND SUPPORT

Follow-up visits are the heartbeat of a patient's success in the program. The initial visit is exposing the patient to the doctor's know-how and attitude of caring for him or her. I have a white board hanging in my office that provides a space to write the patient's plan and illustrate examples. I review the program along with providing tips on how to lose the weight successfully, effectively and safely. A key purpose of the initial consultation is to win the patient's confidence and cultivate trust and loyalty. The first impression creates the patient's willingness to follow the program. A patient must feel comfortable and reassured that his/her physician is going to be with him/her throughout the entire weight loss journey.

A patient's bi-weekly visit can be a most challenging event. This is the time to overcome any objection, any doubt, any negative feeling or thoughts that a patient experiences after the first week on the program. Patients are scheduled for a return visit one week after their initial visit. This second visit provides time to fine-tune the patient's program. It also allows him or her to express how he/she feels about the program, and gives them the desire and determination to pursue more weight loss until a healthy weight is achieved. Most patients lose four or five pounds in one week and thus become excited. Some patients do not lose this much.

Whatever the amount of weight loss, the patient is encouraged to practice patience as his or her body adjusts to a new way of living. When he or she doesn't get immediate results, my question to him/her is, "How much are you willing to do in order to experience success?" I remind the patient that success is a process. It requires patience and a good attitude. "Patience is bitter, but the fruit is sweet," as my father used to say.

Patients can become discouraged during this process. There are reasons why the scales may not show much loss during the follow-up visits. There may be situations arising both at home and at work. Stress can play a large part. Whatever the reason, when they practice persistence, it will reap big rewards.

I discuss priorities with the patient without being judgmental. Counseling, encouragement, reinforcement and motivation are required at this point. Frustration and discouragement is part of the process when doing great things for oneself. These factors will either slow one down, or stop one altogether.

This visit is a period of enriching the patient's feelings and attitude. I tell the patient to focus on the outcome, not on the process. I try to bring the best out in every patient by reminding him or her of a bigger picture: to visualize how he/she will look at his/her ideal healthy weight, and experience the happiness that manifests with the decision he/she made.

It is my mission to ensure the patient that he or she made a correct choice and to continue to motivate him or her even through the most challenging times. As my father once quoted during my medical school days, "Even a snail paced its way to Noah's Ark."

ꙮꙮ

"In my current situation I have an elevated blood pressure, high cholesterol, high blood sugar, acid reflux and I am overweight. I take medications for these conditions and my doctor tells me to lose weight. Can you help me, Dr. Ordonez?"

Take the time to dance
It is the source of youth, source
of mind, and body connection
Take the time to sing….
It is the source of spirit
Take the time to laugh…..
It is the music of the soul
Take the time to think….
It is the source of power.
Take the time to Dream…
It is the road to destiny.
Take the time to pray….
It is the greatest power on earth.
Take the time to believe…
It is the source of energy.
Take the time to read…….
It is the fountain of wisdom.
Take the time to say "I love you" …..
It is a God-given privilege.
Take time to work smart…..
It is the price of success
Take a risk, take a chance…..
It is the source of growth and
happiness.

These are the values by which to live your
life.

Dr. Ernie

II

OBESITY

THE PLAGUE OF THE 21ST CENTURY

"To say that obesity is caused by merely consuming too many calories is like saying that the only cause of the American Revolution was the Boston Tea Party."

Adelle Davis, Nutritionist/Writer
1904-1974

ONE ℘ A MODERN DILEMMA

"Americans will be more likely to change their behavior if they have a meaningful reward—something more than just reaching a certain weight or dress size. The real reward is invigorating, energizing, joyous health. It is a level of health that allows people to embrace each day and live their lives to the fullest without disease or disability."

VADM Regina M. Benjamin, M.D., M.B.A., Surgeon General[6]

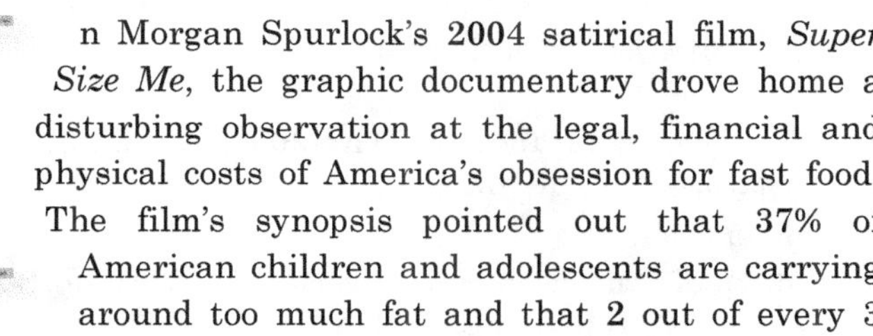

In Morgan Spurlock's 2004 satirical film, *Super Size Me*, the graphic documentary drove home a disturbing observation at the legal, financial and physical costs of America's obsession for fast food. The film's synopsis pointed out that 37% of American children and adolescents are carrying around too much fat and that 2 out of every 3 adults are overweight or obese.[7] The film covered the horror of school lunch programs, the declining programs for health and physical education, food addictions and the exaggerated and dangerous measures individuals take to lose weight.

Overweight is not just an issue in the U.S. Lauren Streb's 2007 article in Forbes Magazine, *World's Fattest Countries*[8], pointed out that in recent studies conducted by the World Health Organization on increased world obesity, smaller countries undergoing economical development that have adopted more Western Lifestyles through urbanization, introduction of fast foods chains, show marked increases in what is called a *nutrition transition*. Smaller countries that once dealt primarily with under nutrition are now fighting obesity.

Each year in the United States, 300,000 people die annually from obesity and overweight, making it the second leading cause of preventable death, behind smoking.[9] Mississippi, Tennessee and Alabama rank the highest in obesity with a gigantic 30% or higher due to increased poverty levels and poor Lifestyle. Colorado has the lowest obesity level in the U.S. between 15%-18%. It boasts a higher level of fitness and Lifestyle.[10]

According to American Sports Data, Inc. the statistics on America's obesity epidemic reports that 3.8 million people in the U.S. weigh over 300 pounds, with 400,000 individuals (mostly males) carry over 400 pounds.[11] The average adult female weighs a record 163 pounds. The National Center for Health statistics[12] reports that

- Between 1962 and the year 2000, the number of obese Americans grew from 13% to an alarming 31% of the population.
- 63% of Americans are overweight with a Body Mass Index (BMI) in excess of 25.0.
- 31% are obese with a BMI in excess of 30.0.

TWO ꕤ ATTITUDES ON OBESITY

Lee and Oliver (2002) conducted a poll to characterize Americans' attitudes about obesity in order to determine how attitudes and beliefs affect support for obesity-related policy changes. They asserted that

> *"the concept of "moral failure" is at the root of public opinions that hold obesity as a personal choice and responsibility. They posited that obesity violates the valued American trait of self-reliance. Characterizing people who are obese as lazy, undisciplined, and lacking self-control enables the public to hold them responsible for their condition, and may be used as justification for bias and discrimination. The authors also posited that when obesity is understood as resulting from a lack of individual*

motivation, there will be little support for such policies as government regulations, civil protections, or taxes to prevent and decrease it.[13]

Additionally, there can be sensitivity when using the term *overweight* with children, as reported by Dr. Daniel Kirschenbaum, Professor of Psychiatry and Behavior Sciences, Northwestern University Medical School and clinical director of Wellspring Academies a leading weight loss camp. A 2002 National Health and Nutrition Examination Survey revealed that only 36.7% of overweight kids had actually been told by a doctor or other health care professional that they were overweight.[14] And here's a frightening fact: Childhood obesity in the United States has more than tripled in the past two decades.

There still may be many people who don't think carrying extra weight is nearly as dangerous as it is. There is an overall denial among 51% of American that this is really an issue. The fact stands undeniably obvious that being overweight and obese can kill you. It increases your risk of developing the following:

- Coronary heart disease
- Type 2 diabetes
- Cancers (endometrial, breast, and colon)
- Hypertension (high blood pressure)
- Dyslipidemia (for example, high total cholesterol or high levels of triglycerides)
- Stroke
- Liver and gallbladder disease
- Sleep apnea and respiratory problems
- Osteoarthritis (a degeneration of cartilage and its underlying bone within a joint)
- Gynecological problems (abnormal menses, infertility)

Obesity is at its highest having reached national epidemic proportions, becoming the mother of all diseases and an index of morbidity and mortality. Obesity becomes the *open door* that gives birth to more disease. More Americans are overweight now than at any other time in our history. The problem is not limited to adults but threatens children of all ages as well. And the lifespan of obese/overweight children are indeed shortened.

Obesity has much to do with a sedentary lifestyle, where children and adults spend more time sitting than walking. Our lifestyle and our environment have allowed this condition of obesity/overweight to increase at an alarming rate and has become a pressing health problem for our nation. Lack of exercise and physical activities results in deposits of excess or unused fat cells, causing obesity. Additionally, managing obese/overweight people is growing into a heavy burden for physicians and the national economy.

Obesity Levels in the U.S.

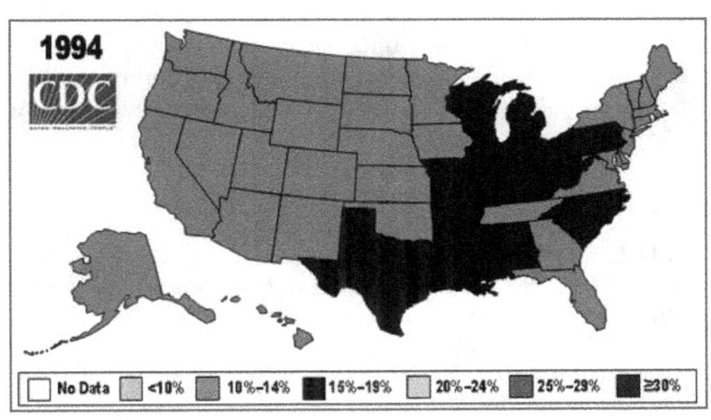

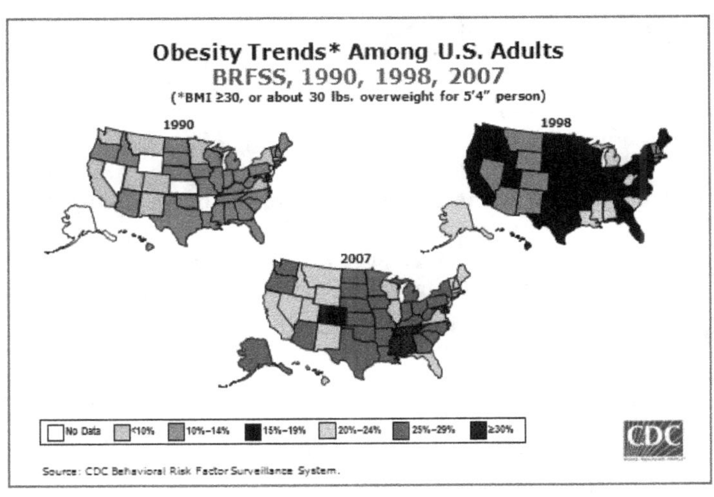

THREE ℘ CHILDHOOD OBESITY

A most disturbing concern is what I have witnessed the last two generations of our children becoming alarmingly over weight and obese. Thirty-one per cent of all adolescents are currently beyond a healthy weight. A recent report stated that this is the first time in history that children may not outlive their parents. Children are developing health issues unheard of 25 years ago. According to the American Academy of Child Adolescent Psychiatry, when one parent is obese, the child has a 50% chance of being overweight. When both parents are obese, this rate creases to 80%. [15,16]

What is also shocking is the adult common disease NAFLD (Non-alcoholic Fatty Liver Disease) now being found in children. Compared to healthy children, a study of 239 children enrolled in the study were found to have poor physical and psychosocial health including being overweight and obese.[17]

While blame can be placed on a medical disorder, the truth is that only 1% is actually caused by physical problems.[18] The REAL reason includes poor eating habits – overeating and binging, lack of exercise, emotional issues and family history of obesity. Physical long-term complications include increased risk of heart disease, diabetes, high blood pressure, breathing issues, and sleep disorders.[19]

Food choices in our school lunch programs have deteriorated to the point that it sends out a deafening alarm stating that our education system is no longer a good role model for health. A study conducted by Davis, Brennan (2002-2005) found that students who had access to fast food restaurant within a half mile of the school ate less fruit and vegetables and were more likely to be overweight. [20] There is a 5% increase in child obesity in a nearby school when a fast food establishment is within walking distance.

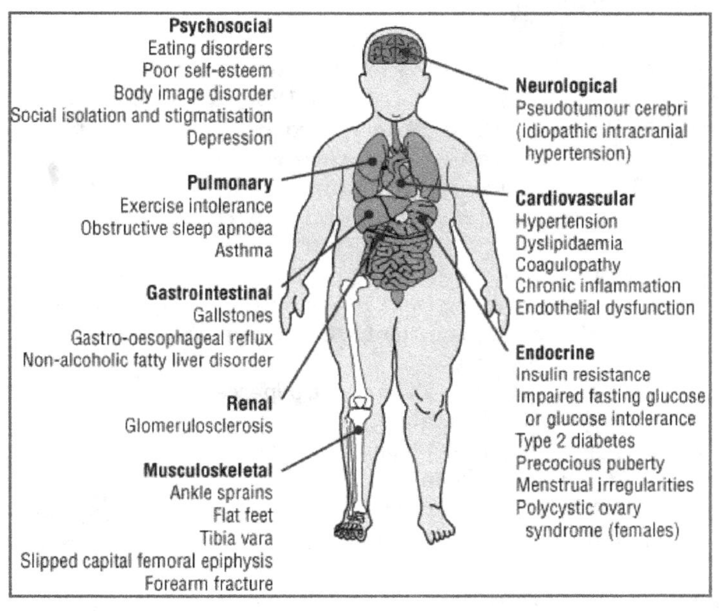
Psychosocial
Eating disorders
Poor self-esteem
Body image disorder
Social isolation and stigmatisation
Depression
Pulmonary
Exercise intolerance
Obstructive sleep apnoea
Asthma
Gastrointestinal
Gallstones
Gastro-oesophageal reflux
Non-alcoholic fatty liver disorder
Renal
Glomerulosclerosis
Musculoskeletal
Ankle sprains
Flat feet
Tibia vara
Slipped capital femoral epiphysis
Forearm fracture
Neurological
Pseudotumour cerebri
(idiopathic intracranial
hypertension)
Cardiovascular
Hypertension
Dyslipidaemia
Coagulopathy
Chronic inflammation
Endothelial dysfunction
Endocrine
Insulin resistance
Impaired fasting glucose
or glucose intolerance
Type 2 diabetes
Precocious puberty
Menstrual irregularities
Polycystic ovary
syndrome (females)

BMI of American Children

Obesity has prevailed in children between the ages of 6 to 11, with an increase of 6.5% in 1980 to 19.6% in 2008. Prevalence in years 12 to 19 increased from 5.0% in 1980 to 19.6% in 2008.[21] According to the American Heart Association, when defining overweight in children and adolescents, it's important to consider both weight and body composition.

Among American children ages 2–19, the following are overweight or obese, using the 95th percentile or higher of body mass index (BMI) values on the CDC 2000 growth chart:

- For non-Hispanic whites, 31.9 percent of males and 29.5 percent of females.
- For non-Hispanic blacks, 30.8 percent of males and 39.2 percent of females.
- For Mexican Americans, 40.8 percent of males and 35.0 percent of females.

The prevalence of overweight (BMI-for-age values at or above the 95th percentile of the 2000 CDC growth charts) in children ages 6–11 increased from 4.0 percent in 1971–74 to 17.0 percent in 2003–06. The prevalence of overweight in adolescents ages 12–19 increased from 6.1 percent to 17.6 percent (NHANES, NCHS).[22]

Child Obesity in the U.S.

Figure 2. Prevalence of obesity among boys aged 12–19 years, by race/ethnicity: United States, 1988–1994 and 2007–2008

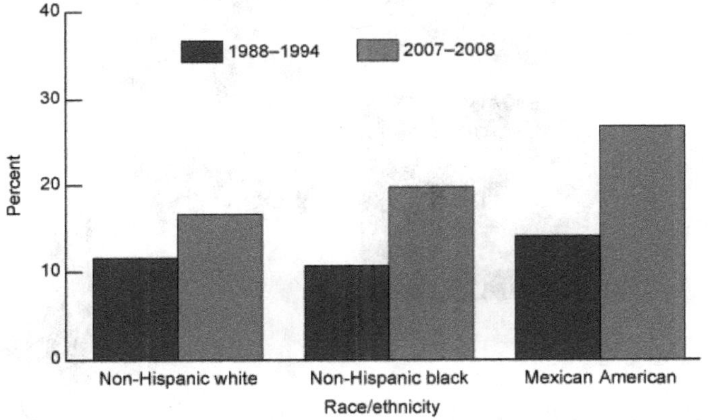

40
30
Percent
20
10
0

1988–1994 2007–2008

Non-Hispanic white Non-Hispanic black Mexican American

Race/ethnicity

NOTE: Obesity is defined as body mass index (BMI) greater than or equal to sex- and age-specific 95th percentile from the 2000 CDC Growth Charts.
SOURCES: CDC/NCHS, National Health and Nutrition Examination Survey (NHANES) III 1988–1994 and NHANES 2007–2008.

Figure 3. Prevalence of obesity among girls aged 12–19 years, by race/ethnicity: United States, 1988–1994 and 2007–2008

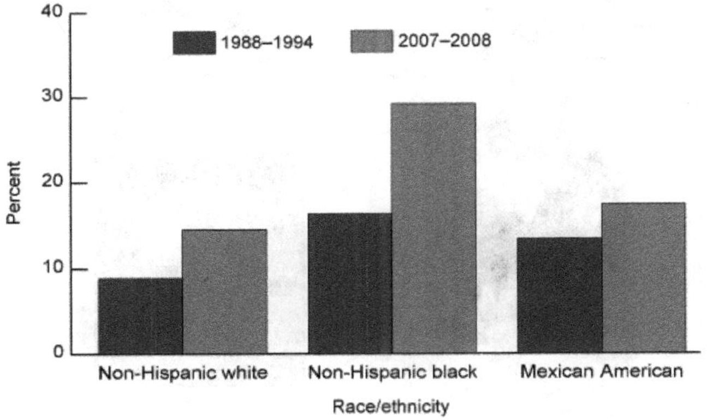

40
30
Percent
20
10
0

1988–1994 2007–2008

Non-Hispanic white Non-Hispanic black Mexican American

Race/ethnicity

NOTE: Obesity is defined as body mass index (BMI) greater than or equal to sex- and age-specific 95th percentile from the 2000 CDC Growth Charts.
SOURCES: CDC/NCHS, National Health and Nutrition Examination Survey (NHANES) III 1988–1994 and NHANES 2007–2008.

Photo Album

Children in the 1950s & '60s

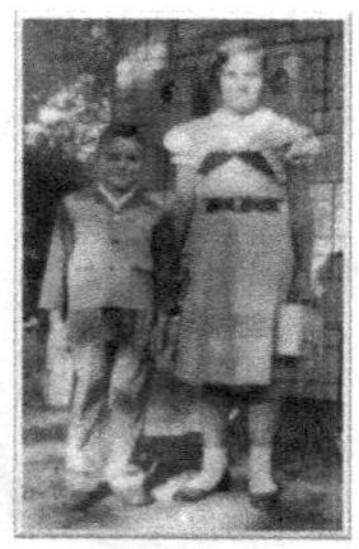

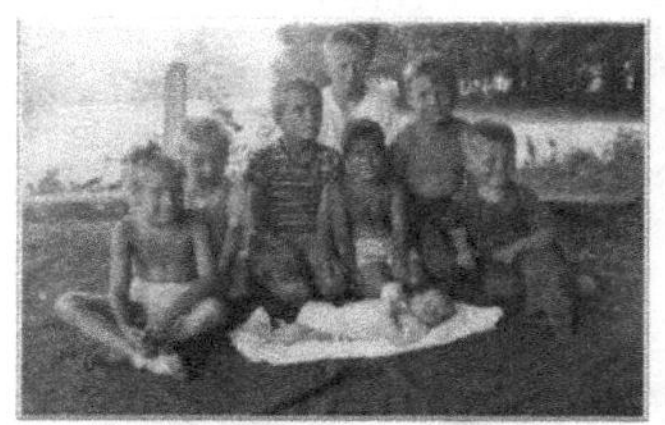

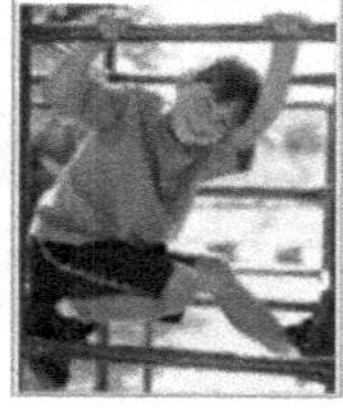

AND NOW……

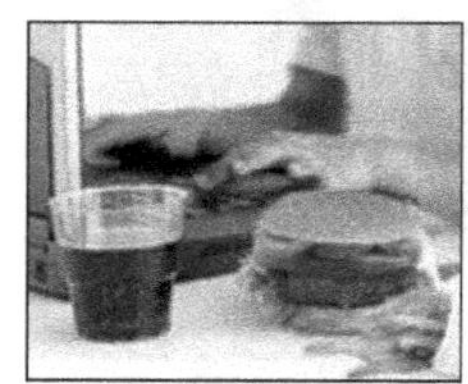

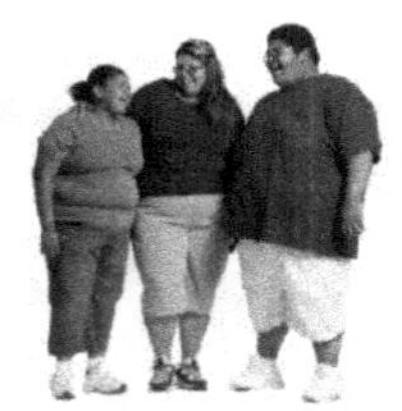

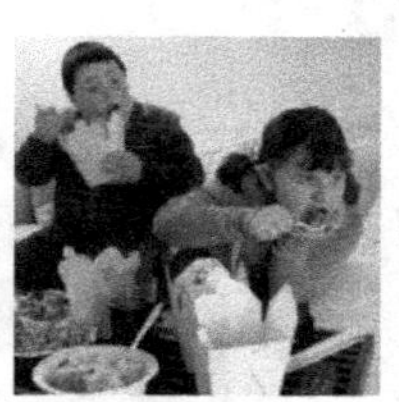

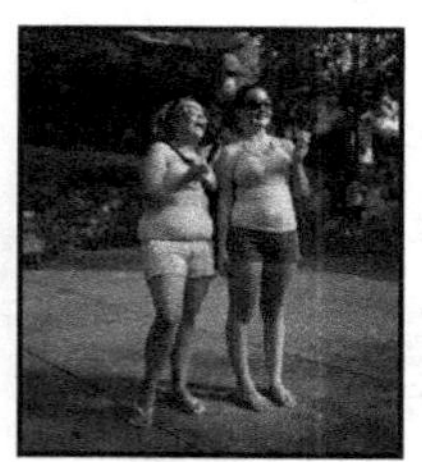

FOUR ꕤ OBESITY AND THE ELDERLY

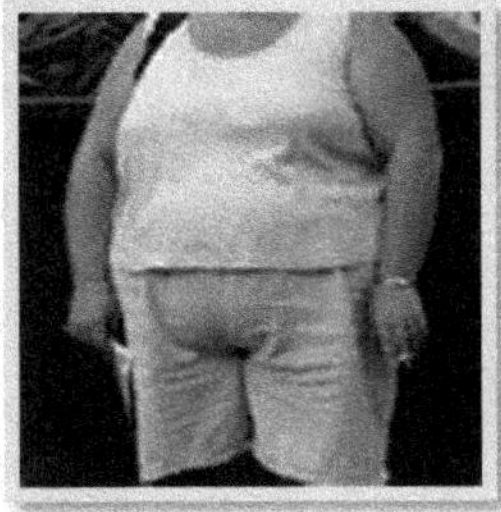

Nearly fifty per cent of the North American population is over **50** years of age and there is growing concern that an increase in obesity will increase the biological aging factors. Moreover, obesity tends to be a global epidemic. University of Australia Leon Flicker, PhD, writes that,

"In industrialized countries, the prevalence of overweight and obesity in older people is a growing public health concern, particularly because sustained again of their populations is expected to continue for many decades, and obesity and aging represent large components of healthcare spending."[23]

Given the current state of the economy, the Baby Boomer generation continues to stay in the work force instead of retiring. They may be still dealing with supporting their children while they attend college. To compound this economic strain, there will be a groundswell of Baby Boomers caring for elder family members. By the year **2050** there will be a significant number of people over **65**. The health care system is already under strain to care for the elderly.[24]

When the elderly experience health challenges, the quality of living and ability to be productive diminishes. Add in an obesity issue and the health risk factors become surreal. Personal medical costs soar along with mitigation of the quality of life. Life becomes a series of interruptions with trips to the doctor and pharmacy and focus on being sick. This pattern consistently reduces a person's quality of living.

Statistics prove that people are healthier and happier when they can lead a normal, happy life filled with activities through social interactions with family and friends.

When there is impaired mobility and chronic ailments, it leads to poor circulation and mental anguish. There is a tremendous mind/body connection that interplays with the well-being of an individual. A feeling of hopelessness, depression, and low self-esteem presents itself when a person is challenged with poor health.

OBESITY RELATED MEDICAL EXPENSES ARE HIGH

Medical spending for treating illnesses and symptoms related to obesity among adults of all ages who live in the community is high, accounting for 5.3 percent of total annual medical expenditures in the United States in 1998, or nearly $27 billion. About half of these expenses are financed by Medicare and Medicaid.[4]

FIGURE 6

Medical Spending Attributable to Obesity for All Adults, by Payer Source

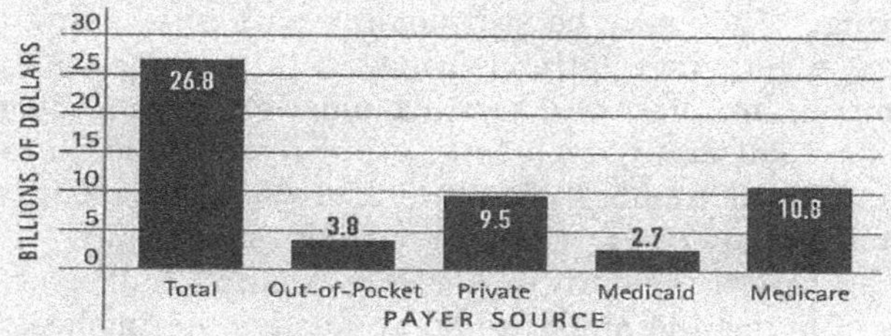

SOURCE: Finkelstein, E.A., Fiebelkorn, I.C. and Wang, G. (2003). National Medical Spending Attributable to Overweight and Obesity: How Much, and Who's Paying? *Health Affairs.* Web Exclusive. Exhibit 4.

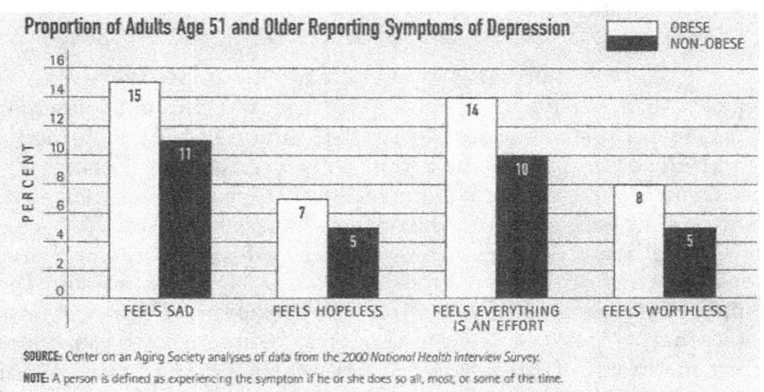

SOURCE: Center on an Aging Society analyses of data from the *2000 National Health Interview Survey.*
NOTE: A person is defined as experiencing the symptom if he or she does so all, most, or some of the time.

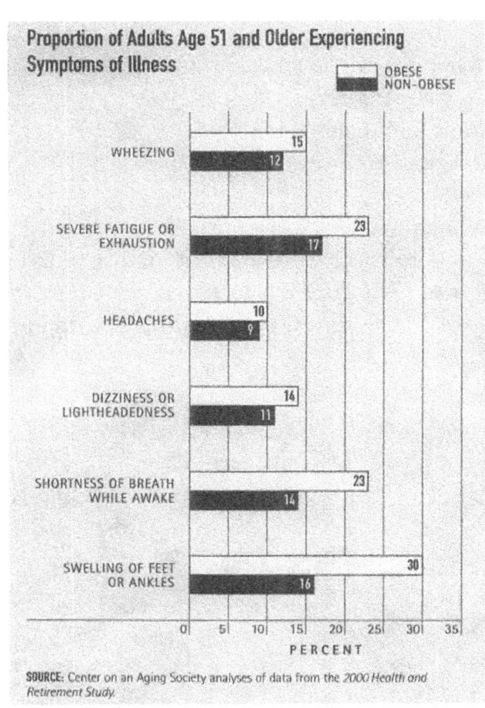

SOURCE: Center on an Aging Society analyses of data from the *2000 Health and Retirement Study.*

(Not) The final word on aging

Advanced progress is being made in almost every area of health. Most far-reaching of all, we are beginning to conquer mankind's worst nemesis — AGING and DEATH. Aging is essentially a process in which your cells lose their resilience; they lose their ability to repair damage. It is in your power, however, to boost that resilience and slow down that process.

Ultimately, our bodies were not designed to fail; they were designed with great efficacy, organization and possess the ability to repair themselves. Michael Brickey, in *Defying Aging*, noted that, when observing modern-day centenarians, there is a common thread of reasons why they reached to be 100. What keeps them young and vital is based on several fundamental traits:[25]

1. They are physically active
2. Few smoke
3. They have maintained a constant weight most of their lives
4. They are mentally alert
5. Self-reliant and independent
6. Optimistic and possess a sense of humor
7. Have good coping skills
8. Don't hold on to losses or resentments

We are able to relish an enhanced quality of living no matter how old we are. We are able to dance long into the night and make love with a body that is alive and filled with desire and life!

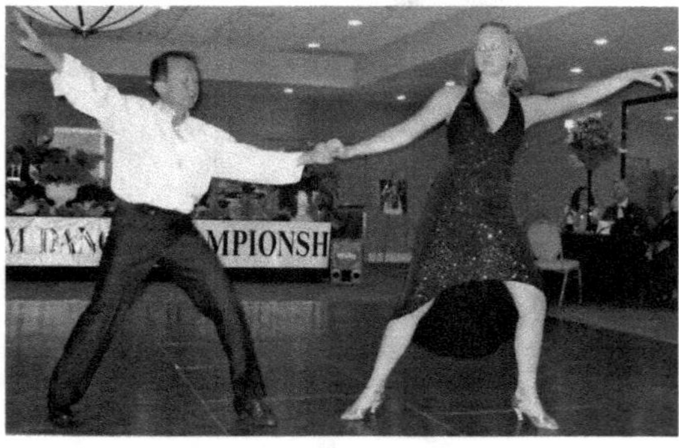

FIVE ഋ DEFINING OBESITY

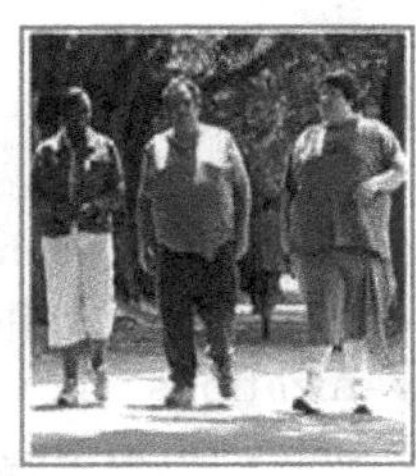

Obesity is a DISEASE....

As such, it is the only disease that is contracted by the WILL, and it is the only disease that requires the WILL to propagate it.

It is the only disease that promotes more diseases - diabetes, hypertension, stroke, gall bladder disease, osteoarthritis, and sleep disorders/apnea, some forms of cancer, depression, stress, incontinence and asthma.

Overweight is a disease that is increased through advertising. Collectively, all of these diseases cause undue suffering, economic hardship, and ultimately — DEATH.

A temporary satisfaction leading to permanent destruction!

Medically, obesity is defined as an excess accumulation of body fat with an increase in size and number of fat cells. Overweight denotes excessive body weight relative to height. The Body Mass Index, or BMI, is the most common medical assessment of obesity and overweight.

Formula: BMI = (Weight/Height squared) X 703

<u>Overweight is defined as a body mass index (BMI) of 25 to 29.9 kg/m^2 to 29.9 kg/m^2 and obesity as a BMI of > 30 kg/m^2.</u> Overweight and obesity are undeniably linked: one can lead to another if a person loses control over his or her body.[26]

Obesity easily leads to metabolic syndrome that is responsible for a host of diseases: hypertension (high blood pressure), diabetes, hyperlipidemia (high fat cell count in the blood) and hyperinsulinemia (high insulin levels in the blood). Since obesity carries a risk of high mortality from all the above causes, it can be called the "weapon of mass extinction".

One of the strongest warnings came from the U.S. Surgeon General, who stated that failure to address overweight and obesity could wipe out some of the gains we've made in areas such as heart disease, several forms of cancer and other chronic health problems. Public health officials and organizations have disseminated health warnings and messages regarding the dangers of obesity but they have not produced the desired effect nationwide.

Pharmaceutical and bio-engineering companies continue their pursuit for the "Magic Bullet".

It has been predicted that costs for obesity is about $344 billion in medical-related expenses by 2018.[27] Studies and results have confirmed that obesity is a major public health problem that appears to lesson life expectancy, especially among individuals in younger age groups. Quality of life is markedly decreased, while suffering is increased.

A Sedentary Lifestyle

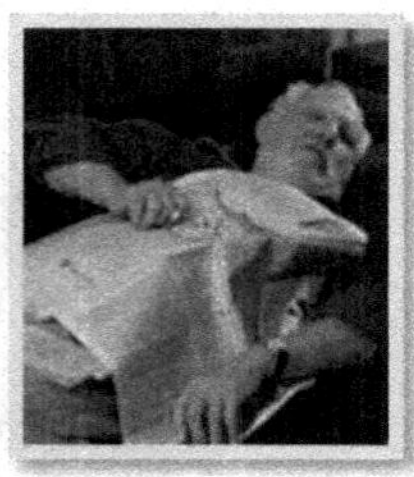

One in ten deaths in the U.S. is associated with a sedentary lifestyle.[28] Chronic health conditions associated with sedentary living contribute to inactivity, which is the third leading cause of premature death in the United States today. Physical inactivity contributes to one of the highest causes of death in the U.S., which is OBESITY. [29]

Clearly, a sedentary lifestyle increases the risk of devastating chronic health conditions and their associated morbidities, leading to human suffering and total loss of quality of life. Dependency on long-term caregivers often leads to deprivation of necessary services and abuse of patients.[30] Being sedentary is also associated with a greater risk of mortality in women than in men.[31]

In 1987, approximately 90 million U.S. inhabitants had one or more chronic health conditions and the population percentage with at least one chronic condition increased with age: 25% in those 18 years and younger; 35% in those 18-44 years old; 68% in those 45 to 64 years old; and 88% in the elderly, those more than 65 years old. Almost 65% of overweight children 5-19 years old already have one bio-clinical or clinical cardiovascular risk factor: elevated blood pressure or increased insulin levels, and 25% have two or more.[32] These risk factors in children are, in part, due to watching more TV and using electronic games and overeating.

Category	**BMI**	**Obesity Class**	**Disease Risk Relative to Weight & Waist Circumference Normal Men: >40in (102cm)**	**WOMEN: <35IN (33CM)**
UNDERWEIGHT	<18.5	-	-	
NORMAL	18.5 – 24.9	-	-	
OVERWEIGHT	25 – 29.9		Increased	High
OBESITY	30 – 34.9 35-39.9	1 2	High Very High	Very High Very High
EXTREME OBESITY	>40	3	Extremely High	Extremely High

By **2009**, these rates had dramatically increased, to where health costs are $1.3 trillion/year in the U.S. A rough approximation is that physical inactivity accounts for approximately 15% of the U.S. health care budget, which is approximately **100** billion dollars annually.

Social and Economic Influences

It is reported that a person's health and the likelihood to become ill and have premature death are highly influenced by prevailing social factors such as poor education, low income, and the quality of neighborhood environments. Poor Americans are three times more likely to suffer physical limitations from a chronic illness compared with upper middle-class incomes. Life expectancy for middle-class Americans is six years longer than those who are poor. [33]

Heart Disease

Over one million Americans die of this disease each year = 42% of all deaths. Cardio vascular disease is the leading cause of death for all Americans 35 years of age and older – not limited to the elderly. Heart disease and stroke account for almost 6 million hospitalizations per year. Estimated cost of cardiovascular disease is more than $300 billion annually.[34]

In the March **2006** report in the *Journal of Clinical Investigation on Obesity*, ***PPARδ: a dagger in the heart of the metabolic syndrome***[35] summarized this dilemma in the following:

"Obesity is a growing threat to global health by virtue of its association with insulin resistance, glucose intolerance, hypertension, and dyslipidemia, collectively known as the metabolic syndrome or syndrome X. The nuclear receptors PPARα

and PPARγ are therapeutic targets for hypertriglyceridemia and insulin resistance, respectively, and drugs that modulate these receptors are currently in clinical use. More recent work on the less-described PPAR isotype PPARδ has uncovered a dual benefit for both hypertriglyceridemia and insulin resistance, highlighting the broad potential of PPARδ in the treatment of metabolic disease. PPARδ enhances fatty acid catabolism and energy uncoupling in adipose tissue and muscle, and it suppresses macrophage-derived inflammation. Its combined activities in these and other tissues make it a multifaceted therapeutic target for the metabolic syndrome with the potential to control weight gain, enhance physical endurance, improve insulin sensitivity, and ameliorate atherosclerosis."

Diabetes

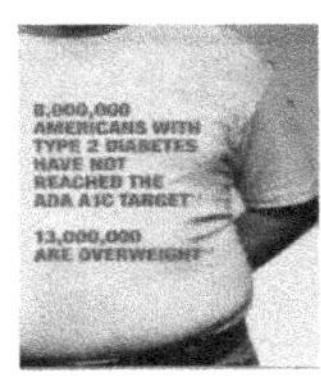

Out of the 44 million American considered obese, 17 million have diabetes.[36] Other study results found that African Americans had the highest rates of obesity (31.1 percent) and diabetes (11.2 percent) compared with other ethnic groups. People with less than a high school education had higher rates of both obesity (27.4 percent) and diabetes (13 percent) than people who had a high school education (Behavioral Risk Factor Surveillance System BRFSS).

In my weight loss practice, we have been able to greatly reduce the diabetic risk factor through weight loss. In diabetes II, a reduction of weight meant a major change in this condition. In several cases, we were able to reduce the amount of daily insulin medication.

Indeed, obesity is already associated with greater morbidity and a poorer health-related quality of life than are smoking, alcoholism or poverty. Despite this, overweight and obesity have not received the same attention from clinicians, health insurance companies, Medicare, Medicaid and policy makers, as have other threats to health such as tobacco use, hypertension, high cholesterol, diabetes and cancers.

It's not surprising that obesity rates continue to climb due to lack of support and participation by these groups. Despite the use of modern medicine in treatments for diseases like hypertension, diabetes, stroke and many forms of cancer and for some chronic health problems like arthritis, the cost, the risks, and the outcome do not change. They continue to rise as Americans become more obese, becoming a disease of the century and a very worrisome epidemic in U.S. history.

80 03

III

NURTURING YOUR LIFE

*"Our current healthcare system is a 'sick care' system with perverse incentives. The disease and economic burden that we have upon us – we currently spend more than $2 trillion per year on health care, or **16%** of our gross domestic product – is largely preventable."*

Richard Carmona, M.D. Chairperson of Partnership to Fight Chronic Disease,
Former Surgeon General 2002-2006

ﻌﻌ

ONE ℘ BURGER AND FRIES

"Nutrition...has been kicked around like a puppy that cannot take care of itself. Food faddists and crackpots have kicked it pretty cruelly."

"We are indeed much more than what we eat, but what we eat can nevertheless help us to be much more than what we are." [37]

Adele Davis, Author, Nutritionist/Writer 1904-1974

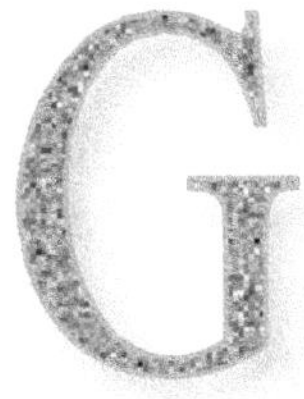

rowing up in Manila, I ate a diet consisting of fish, rice, beans, fruits, nuts, and locally raised meats and produce. Philippine cuisine evolved over several centuries from its Malaysian (Southeast Asian) roots and was vastly influenced by Arab, Indian, Chinese, Japanese, Spanish and American cultures. Throughout the rigors of medical school in Manila, we still ate our native foods.

Medical school provided little education explaining the relationship between nutrition and sickness. Lifestyle factors were not always considered when treating illness. The focus was on treating diseases and not their actual causes. While we studied all the symptoms and knew how to prescribe drugs, we did not have a complete understanding as to the other mind/body aspects of disease.

During April of 1964, I completed medical school and relocated to America. I became a resident in a midwestern hospital located in the birthplace of the American football, Canton, Ohio. The long, exhausting hours of being a resident also brought with it little time to eat healthy food. We ate quickly and chose food that could be consumed in a small amount of time. Consequently, my diet dramatically changed. I was a foreigner in a new country adapting to a new language, new culture, and was exposed to a strange new cuisine called "American fast food." I began consuming fried chicken, hamburgers, pizza, processed foods and many rations that were totally foreign to my body. Late nights found a group of us residents frequenting a local pizza parlor where we decompressed by drinking beer and eating pizza.

It wasn't long before I began to feel dreadful. My biggest surprise came the morning I stepped onto the scales to discover that I had gained a whopping 33 pounds in just three months! My 97-pound body quickly transformed into 130 pounds on a 5'4" frame. My cholesterol went up to 450, triglycerides 800, and sugar levels to 250!

Upon completion of my residency, I relocated to Jacksonville, Florida in the mid 1970s, and joined the medical and hospital community here. I practiced family medicine and general surgery. And of course, I continued eating fast foods and other "not-so-healthy fare".

These habits were quickly corrected when I began to notice patterns in recovery rates of my patients from their illnesses and/or surgery. Weight issues directly correlated to their recovery rates. Some even died due to the complications arising from their poor immune system caused from the stress of increased weight. That obervation influenced the direction of my future.

It meant hours of research, patient observation, and continual investigation as to why they got sick in the first place.

TWO ଔ ONE WITH LIFE

It seems appropriate in this chapter to review the state of our food and the global happenings that lead back to and reflect on our relationship with the planet, the body, and the food sources that sustain us. So what does all of this have to do with obesity?

There is a growing compilation of research and documentaries that demonstrate the global effect regarding the quality of human health and nutrition and the way we view our relationship with food.

Ultimately, this information sheds some light on why we continue to miss the point when it comes to our health and obesity issues. Since the advent of agriculture ten thousand years ago, mankind has been plagued with nutritional deficiencies and disease. We cannot separate our environment, our daily choices, and our human mind, body, or spirit — THEY ARE ONE.

Body By Natural Design

Understanding our genetic relationship between whole, natural foods vs, those that have been genetically altered, refined, or enhanced with colorants or artificial ingredients, is a study in itself.

Our DNA coding for our biological survival was determined over fifty thousand years ago with the dietary habits of hunters and gatherers. Nutrients were taken from unrefined and unprocessed sources of food. The body was designed to recognize and process nutrients through its unique biological sensors and methodology of breaking down the natural foods that it consumed. Enter the 20th Century! Indeed the body was not prepared for the burgers, pizza, soft drinks, refined foods, and fries found in our frenetic modern day diet and Lifestyle.

A few pioneers of the 20th Century began to map the connections between health and food sources. While their observations at the time were frowned upon or thought to be nothing but mere quackery by many in the scientific community, we now realize that these earlier researchers were not so far off the track. Their theories indeed proved to be correct, as we continue to witness the decline of our health, including the rise of obesity and its effect on personal well-being.

Pollan[38] and Byrnes[39] make reference to the studies of Canadian dentist, Weston A. Price, during the 1920s and 1930s. Price studied the relationship between tooth decay, degenerative disease, and diet. His curiosity prompted him to travel to countries investigating the native dietary habits of healthy, nonindustrialized people before they disappeared from the population or were introduced to the Western diet. He noted the relationship between local health and what people ate. Price analyzed the nutrient content of food from one region to another sending samples back to his laboratory. He also took pictures of teeth. He found that isolated populations (primitive races) eating a wide variety of traditional diets were free of dental decay. [40]

Additionally, Price paralled his studies with other observations. He noted the quality of individual health in each region and the effects of the local food they consumed. Was there a difference in health if they ate more animal products and grains, or both? What he discovered was that those who consumed vegetarian and animal foods and fats appeared to be the healthiest. He also noted that those peoples who consumed more grains and legumes suffered from higher rates of dental decay than those who consumed more animal products.

Price's research also concluded that the diet that supports good health is in all respects the very opposite of the dietary recommendations sometimes given by modern day mainstream *health experts*.[41] Once a Western diet was introduced, the signs of tooth decay and degeneration manifested into the population.

So what issues contributed to modern day health issues? It appears that it was the *industrializaton* of our food sources, especially after World War II, that made the difference. The transition from largely agrarian to industrialized methods of food preparation seems to be the real culprit. Moreover, adding in the impact of modern Lifestyles has by far contributed to an increase in chronic diseases.[42] The consumption of refined flour, sugar, canned and chemically preserved foods, and vegetable oils, coupled with a poor Lifestyle have collectively contributed to modern day degenerative disease.[43]

It is difficult to blame any one theory; it is more accurate to imply that it is the collective presence of many influences that has contributed to our present day quandary. While the body has an amazing ability to cope with many foreign substances, it's the amount and frequency of processed foods, artificial ingredients, and frenetic lifestyle (stress) that finally pushes its repair mechanisms beyond the point of no return.

Recognizable Pathways

So what are the biological connections within our body when we eat food that is unrefined and unprocessed versus that which is processed? Let's follow the journey of a fresh peach.

Innate body signals communicate to enzymes and other digstive chemicals when we first touch and smell such a succulent food. This cascade of recognizable events begins through our chemical sensors found in our olfactory system (nose) sending off signals to our brain.[44] As we bite into the fruit, the taste buds in our tongue are able to detect the presence of sweet, salty, sour, bitter, astringent, and umami[45] (glutamate [amino acid] receptors) triggered by the amino acids in foods. These flavors are the smell of *gases* released by the chemicals you've just put in your mouth. Ninety percent of food taste are dependent upon those aromas. And this is also why advertising spends a lot of time and money promoting the succulence and smell of a hamburger in late night TV watching!

The sense of taste has been purported by scientists to be an innate safety mechanism or way of letting us know if we have been poisoned. When the body ingests natural food, it recognizes it and comfortably takes advantage of its entire nutritional value, including the enzymes that assist the digestion in your digestive tract. The consumption of an untainted (unprocessed) food sets up a cascade of accurate reactions in our body that support our cells and body systems as the food is processed throughout the entire digestive system. The plethora of vitamins and minerals originally present in the fruit enter into our system. The fresher it is, the more available nutrients there are.

In contrast, when biting into a food containing artificial flavoring, fragrance, color, artifical sweetener(s), and refined ingredients, these unnatural chemicals emit questionable signals. Processing foods reduces them of vital nutrients, including vitamins.

During a landmark study, the Iowa Women's Health Study[46],[47] (1986 to 2004), the relation of whole-grain versus refined grain consumption was explored. The question arose investigating whether grain fiber or the phytochemicals that coexist with fiber are more important in health? [48] Clinical researchers Jacobs and Steffen state that

"the interrelation of human physiology and of the biological activity of plant and animals foods that humans consume is incredibly complex, replete with checks, balances, and feeback loops, dependent on a myriad of substances that differ only in subtle ways from one another." ...."it is likely that there are additive or more than additive influences of foods and food

constituents on health – that is, food synergy....though the extent and nature of that synergy are different."[49]

Inherently the body may struggle with understanding the authenticity of the chemical composition of foreign components, especially because they often are not metabolized. The refining process also strips the original item of its nutrients. It may smell and taste like the real thing, fooling the senses to a certain degree. The body may be at a loss as to how to handle them. At best, it reluctantly accepts what was eaten, synthesizing less than quality nutrition. These artificial components also add burdens onto the digestive system. How much can the body tolerate, however? It is not surprising to disover why the body no longer copes with the refinement or alteration of food. It can easily end up suffering from allergies, poor digestion, and other ailments.

House of Bandits

In the pursuit of progress, are we robbing ourselves of vital nutrients?

The jury is still out as to fully understanding the long term effects of genetically engineered foods that have been on our supermarket shelves since the mid 1990s. Many plants are genetically modified to increase their resistance to insects and disease, as well as grow faster with higher yields. It is obvious that there is legitimacy in improving agriculture, especially in regions where the technology warrants ingenuity in growing crops. More than sixty percent of all processed foods in the U.S. contain ingredients made from bioengineered soybeans, corn, or canola — ice cream, pizza, corn chips, salad dressing, cookies, baking powder.[50] The question is, what are the long term effects for this?

There is little scientific data concerning the long term health risks of GMOs and what has been published to date.[51,52] The question herein is whether modified and unmodified plants are substantially equivalent once their DNA has been modified. The CFS (Center for Food Safety) has been petitioning the FDA for pre-market testing of GMO food allergens.[53] Testing methods require radical improvement.

Another recent study published by the International Journal of Biological Sciences[54] points out the importance of studying the potential of mid- and long-term toxicological effects during regulatory tests prior to commercialization of chemicals.

Consultant and biochemist, Arpad Pusztai, Ph.D. has pioneered research for the past thirty years into the effects of dietary lectins (carbohydrate-reactive proteins) on the gastro-intestinal tract, including those transgenically expressed in genetically modified crop plants.[55]

A statement from Pollan clearly summarizes several thoughts *"...long familiarity between foods and their eaters leads to elaborate systems of communication up and down the food chain so that a creature's senses come to recognize foods as suitable by their taste and smell and color."* He also asks, *"What would happened if we were to start thinking about food as less of a thing and more of a relationship?"*[56]

As a physician, I continue to discover how optimum body health and longevity require a more profound relationship with ALL that nourishes it: our relationshps, the air, the water, the soil, the plants, and the creatures that give up their life so that we can have food on our tables.

A lesson from early American Indian people showed a great reverence for Mother Earth and all the inhabitants that lived for the benefit of the other. All life is created from the same Source and thus each is honored and loved from the energy from which it is created. Take nothing that we don't require, waste nothing, and offer thanks for everything that sustains us.

The future of our planet is the responsibility of each of us. Having a healthy mind and body ensures that we make good decisions for our future and live our life with vitality and maximum health. Keep that thought deep in your heart.

THREE ꟸ THE EARLY YEARS

Our relationship with the power of food begins in the womb. Whatever our mother consumed, the state of her health including her thoughts, directly affected the quality of our development. When we suckled at the breast or bottle it was a time of nurturing both to our body and our mind. It provided opportune moments to create a deep human bonding with another human being — our mother.

As a young child, our eating habits began to form in the high chair, where we joined the social order of family eating. Future habits are closely tied to the way in which we learned to understand the importance of a balanced (or not-so-balanced) diet. We explored colors and texture and had no inhibition to play with the different shapes that soared in our imaginations. It was fun converting the oatmeal bowl into a hat. We may also recall the hours spent with our Mom and/or Dad in food preparation and the family gathering at the holiday table.

Not so long ago, it was common to have at least two to three meals at home; this provided important family time together, even if for a short while. Down through the ages, eating together nourished not only the body but the soul. Many references are found in literature about "breaking bread together". Numerous cultures consider it a very special time for family interaction.

There were also certain etiquette observances that taught us good manners. While this may vary from culture to culture, many of us remember that we could not leave the table without permission or until everyone was finished.

There were no cell phone interruptions and if the house phone did ring, the caller could not interrupt this personal family time.

Nutrition researcher, food historian, and author Sally Fallon Morrell, MA[57], founding president of the Weston A. Price Foundation for Wise Tradtions in Food, Farming, and the Healing Arts, spoke of this time so eloquently in her presentation at the annual conference of Consumer Health of Canada, March 2002.[58] While she references women, her quote is applicable to all who perform this important charge.

> *"If a woman could see the sparks of light going forth from her fingertips when she is cooking, and the substance of light that goes into the food she handles, she would be amazed to see how much of herself she charges into the meals that she prepares for her family and friends. It is one of the most important and least understood activities of life; the radiation and feeling that go into the preparation of food affect everyone who partakes of it. And this activity should be unhurried, peaceful and happy because the substance of the life stream performing the service flows into that food and is eaten, and actually becomes part of the energy of the receiver."*
>
> *"That substance starts with the way we farm—the farmer that farms with wisdom and love for the land, the dairyman that farms with love for his animals, the cheese maker who makes the cheese with the love of her craft, the baker*

> *who bakes with the love of the final product, the beverage maker who makes the type of delicious and nutritious beverage that I would like to see come to this nation. That energy goes into the food and when it is eaten by the receiver actually blesses the receiver."*

The Single Parent Family

During the later part of the 20th Century, the family unit changed dramatically when both parents were forced to work in order to meet expenses. What compounded the complexity of the family unit was an increase in households headed by a single parent — 12.9 million of them as of 2006; 10.4 million single-mother families and 2.5 million single-father familes.[59]

Packaged meals and convenience foods become common. Shorter preparation time means that we continue to alter our relationship with food, along with the time spent as a family. And finally, some children go to school hungry.

Social Determinants of Health

There are different social factors that are also contributors, such as health literacy, inaccess to healthy foods, resource-poor communities and food deserts. Many inner city neighborhoods are sprinkled with convenience stores, but not large chain stores that provide enough variety. The same holds true for very poor, rural areas throughout many U.S. regions. Health illiteracy issues increase with the inability to understand ingredients on food labels. This could be attributed to a language barrier or the inability to read proficiently, or at all. Even greater is the lack of a fundamental understanding of nutrition and how to make a healthy choice when it comes to food. Given the low overall illiteracy rate in this country, 21-23% or 40-44 million people,[60] health literacy is exacerbated by this situation. Hitting the pocketbook hard, healthy foods cost more. Poor income families just cannot afford them.[61] When people are homeless, they go into nutritional deficiency, affecting their thinking, behavior, and ability to have quality of life. [62]

Media Craze - Diet Foolish

Individuals tend to listen to TV ads instead of really understanding what it is to read a food label. Watching TV has brainwashed us into thinking we're hungry when we're not. The tendency is to reach for what is familiar and convenient such as what is seen advertised for fast food chains.

Current diet crazes have estranged us in how we value our own thoughts on food and our body. Instead of choosing quality food as a nurturing necessity, we over-consume by eating refined foods that "taste good"and are filling, but lower in nutritional benefits.

Modern supermarket foods don't always appear like the foods that grandmother made. She would be baffled when choosing from such a hodgepodge of strange packaging and imitation products that is called "food".

It is very common practice to eat so quickly that our brain has little time to register its relevance. Additionally, food becomes a platform for guilt when we think we're eating something that is "bad" for us. "Eating on the run" has contributed to poor food choices, overeating, and poor digestion. It is time to reconsider how we are going to alter our relationship with food so that it becomes a positive experience with a healthy outcome.

FOUR ☙ FOOD PROFITS — A LINK TO OBESITY

The 21st Century shopping environment has moved a long way from small general country store settings with bins of flour, sugar, fresh bakery items, local meats, produce and dry goods. Currently, the grocery industry spends millions of dollars annually to transform our shopping experience into a gastronomic milieu with mounds of displays and neatly wrapped containers of meat, fish, produce, dairy and other exotic specialty imports in multiple varieties made possible by modern preservation and shipping methods. They also supply quick-fix microwave meals and processed food stuff. Modern transport methods make possible the purchase of groceries from across North America and countries outside of the U.S. such as South America, Asia and Europe.

The amount of crop yields produced in the United States is now the highest in history. It is not surprising that this abundance not only feeds Americans, but also many people throughout the world. Yet this overproduction still does not reach remote global areas, including some in the U.S., where hunger becomes a daily occurance.

In America, this enormous food yield influences how it is promoted, with greater focus on the way people eat. There is a deluge of super-sized consumption and a continuous torrent of ready snacks throughout the day.

Gigantic marketing and advertising capaigns cleverly display everything from cereals, toilet paper, toothpaste, and meat, to canned goods, coffee, teas, confection, and processed foods. Manufacturers pay for positioning on store shelves to obtain direct eye attention of passing by shoppers, including children. Sugar-coated cereals are placed at eye level for the child sitting in the shopping cart seat.[63] Additional artificial coloring is placed in foods such as cereals to entice younger children. The FDA has now released studies linking artificial food dyes to hyperactivity in children.[64] An astonishing 34+ billion dollars a year are spent by the food industry to advertise their products. Twelve billion dollars are spent on commercials directed toward children, who watch more than **10,000** food messages a year.[65]

Competition is high among food manufacturers. Along with the advertising are the millions of research dollars spent to establish new theories about re-designing foods that are already highly processed in order to make them even more appealing to the consumer. Notice the increase of "buzz", words found on packaging and labels — "fortified with antioxidants", "low fat", "omega-3's", "low carbohydrates". What better way to sell a product, than by including terminology on packaging that helps to get it quickly into our shopping cart. What is listed on the box may be true; however, the real question arises in how much, and what source? Is a processed food really healthy?

At the Children's Hospital and Research Center in Berkeley, California, senior scientist and biomedical researcher, Bruce Ames and his research team study possible cancer hazards from human exposure to chemicals, including food additives, air pollutants and pesticides. They found that even subtle nutrient deficiencies cause DNA damage, which eventually leads to cancer. [66] When starved of vital nutrients, an individual will continue to eat in order to feel satiated. This is yet one more argument to alter our eating habits so that we don't undermine our own ability to lose weight.

Given the amount of subsidies paid annually, it is interesting to note which foods receive the highest attention. Subsidies also make these foods more affordable. Approximately **90%** of all subsidies support just five crops — wheat, cotton, corn, soybeans, rice — while fruits and vegetables receive very little [67,68].

What is more remarkable are the enormous profits that have seeped over into the drug industry from the promotion of meat, dairy and fast foods. Billions of dollars go into research to create medication to treat the diseases that unfold from poor eating habits. There is much more profit from developing new drugs than in placing a larger focus on prevention.

This further accounts for the growing concern regarding the effect of promotion and its contribution to the ever mounting obesity issue.

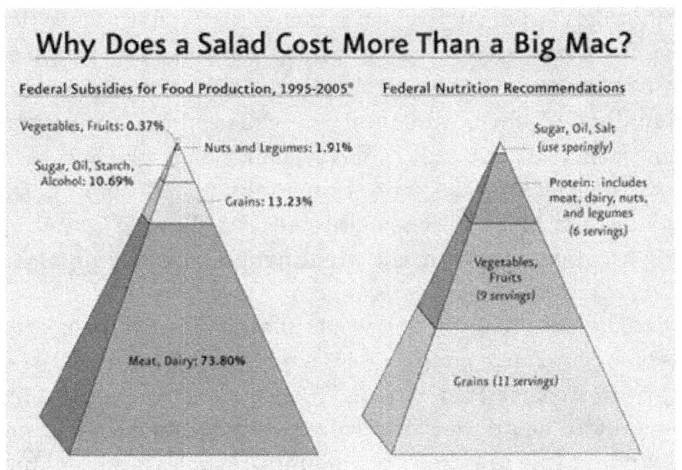

FIVE ☙ THE NEW FARM

The nature of traditional farming has changed rapidly during the latter part of the past century, and so has the way we eat and consume on a daily basis. Fewer cattle and other animals graze leisurely in open, green pastures. The small American farm is just about extinct as it is replaced with large commerical "farming" methods to meet the demands for beef for the fast food industry and general consumption. Cattle are placed in crowded feed lots where they are fed a diet of corn instead of grass. This forces them to grow fast. Hogs and poultry are not exempt from this method of mass production. Animals dwelling in tight living situations causes them to become diseased and experience abnormal stress. Thus they are given antibiotics to keep them "healthy", along with growth hormones, to make them grow faster. There is a vast difference in animal behavior while growing on rangeland or pastures, and in corrals. They instinctively respond to their surroundings, especially when it comes to predators. When moved from range to corral, animals require conditioning to their new surroundings so that they don't feel threatened. Mishandling of farm animals can cause them to become traumatized. It not only affects their behavior, but their ability to resist disease, and ultimately is reflected in the quality of their meat, once slaughtered. Dr. Temple Grandin's ground-breaking work in the treatment of farm animals is worth reading.[69]

The fast food industry has placed huge demands on farmers for beef and poultry.[70] Fifty percent of all raised beef are grown for fast food chains.[71] Americans are consuming excess protein at an alarming rate — all too much. And not withstanding this are the vast amounts of cholesterol-building fats that are consumed at the same time, making heart disease and related ailments to be at an all time record high.

SIX ☙ DEPLETING SOILS

Non-organic produce is grown in soils that are conditioned with pesticides and industrial fertilizers that biologically simplify soil chemistry. They also affect the biological activity of the soil's underground ecosystem, destroying valuable soil microbes, soil enzymes, earthworms and mycorrhizal fungi. Eventually the ground becomes depleted of its natural minerals, forcing plants to sacrifice their own enzymes to replenish the soil in which they grow. University of Illinois researchers Mulvaney, Khan, and Ellsworth argue that the "net effect of nitrogen use is to reduce soil's organic matter content....nitrogen fertilizer stimulates soil matter which feast on organic matter. Over time, the impact of this enhanced microbial appetite outweighs the benefits of nitrogen residues."[72]

Plants are genetically engineered in order to produce higher yields with greater resistance to disease. A bean plant of 40 years ago has been transformed into a hardier bean that defies pests and disease, giving a higher yield in less growth time. What about its nutritional value?

Commercial farming includes the use of synthetic fertilizers and pesticides and sometimes inappropriate crop rotation. These practices are leading to the depletion of precious soil minerals and other nutrients. In order for plants to receive higher soil nutrients, they need to develop deep root systems and remain in the ground for a longer duration. Faster production means that root systems are shallow and do not spend a lot of time taking in these vital components.

While there may be argument justifying modern methods, the bottom line may be to explore whether we are ingesting more than just a pure vegetable, meat or fruit.

SEVEN ☙ THE BEEF BEHIND THE BURGER

Not only are we growing and consuming an excess amount of protein, we are increasing the use of pesticides on crops consumed by farm animals. These end up in the animals' tissues and fat, and include the growth hormones that were consumed when they were alive. Eventually, they show up on our dinner plate. The U.S. produced 12.9 million tons of beef in 2008.[73] Annually, the American consumption of beef averages about 67.1 pounds per person.[74] Not surprisingly, American beef has been banned in many European Union countries, as well as in Asian countries.[75] While there is argument concerning these practices when it comes to producing meat, there is a large question as to its actual effect on overall health. Are they trying to tell us something?

Prior to 1948, there was little heart disease. It is now a #1 killer, with cancer close behind. Prior to 1948, our diet was based on consuming more plant-based foods since the cost of meat was high and therefore reserved for the upper class As beef became more readily affordable, the demands for it increased. Eating has become the biggest cause of two out of three deaths in the U.S. What the statistics prove is that when a society moves from a plant-based diet to one of animals, we end up with increased arterial diseases that cause poor circulation. Combine a sedentary lifestyle with that, and the outcome is disastrous.

What has happened to our food is killing us. According to recent statistics, including my own observations over the years, 70-85 percent of all hospital patients become heir to illnesses associated with diet-induced diseases. The promotion of fast foods, diet drinks, artificial sugars, abundance of high fructose corn syrup, artificial colorants and highly processed food has brought in millions of dollars to producers and manufacturers. Heavy advertising has tricked our minds into believing that unless the label says low fat, sugar free, low calorie, we should not buy a product. Sadly, poor eating habits during the past 30 years have contributed to a pandemic of obesity that is leading to our having less-resistant immune systems, disease and death.

EIGHT ☙ LAND TO SEA

Oceans cover 70% of the earth. Ninety per cent of the earth's oxygen is produced through the photosynthesis of phytoplankton and sea algae.[76] There is growing concern for their future as they become more polluted and overfished.

In a 2006 ABC National Radio documentary, The Rising Tide of Ocean Plagues,[77] scientists voiced their concerns about the state of the world's oceans and coral reefs: the effects of aquaculture on wild fish populations; disease in sea creatures and how coral reefs are being lost due to over-fishing, global warming and pollution. Humans have used these precious waters for dumping grounds leaving millions of pounds of trash including plastic, which takes about 1000 years to decompose. Thousands of whales, birds, seals and turtles are killed every year from plastic litter since they mistake them for food. The results are devastating. We are killing off our own food sources in our drive for convenience and high yield. It's like sweeping the dirt under the rug, ignoring the very life that sustains us.

When we become negligent toward our own surroundings, it isn't long before a cascade of destructive and alarming events becomes apparent. Suddenly, we realize that in the end we are harming and degrading our own body and quality of life. It cannot always cope with the "foreign" additives found in our food such as flavor enhancers and artificial colors and refined ingredients.

Injecting artificial food coloring into the flesh of farm-raised salmon is a common practice in order to give their flesh a pink color.[78] Wild pink salmon obtain their natural pink/orange color from a fat soluble carotenoid pigment called astaxanthin taken from their diet. It is found in marine algae, zooplankton and krill. Astaxanthin is a natural anti-oxidant found in the fish and is considered ten times more effective as an antioxidant than other carotenoids, and one hundred times more powerful than vitamin E.

NINE ☙ TIMELESS TRADITION — HEALTHY LIFE

For centuries, many cultures consumed 5% of animal foods and 95% of whole plant foods. In countries where there is a hunter-gatherer population, such as in New Guinea, they traditionally eat more than 800 varieties of plant food. Americans consume fewer than 20 fruits and vegetables. The Western world consumes 42% of animal foods, 51% of refined foods and 7% of whole plant foods.

Historically, populations who consume higher levels of meat are destined for diseases such as heart disease. Countries deemed "poor" may actually be healthier because of the simple foods that they consume. Many follow a traditional whole plant food diet that has not been influenced by the diet of the Western world (Pollen, 2007).[79]

In his recent book, *Blue Zones*, Dan Buettner and his team of scientists studied five different areas of the world where the local population lives the longest and are the healthiest.[80] These areas include Sardinia, Italy, where there are 20 times more centarians than in the United States. Northern Costa Rica boasts some of the longest-lived and healthiest people in the world. Buettner and his team concluded that the biggest controllable factor for longevity and health is where we live — not education, marital status and wealth. His *Power9* concepts indicate that making changes to your environment promotes changes within your life. They include nine behaviors that will influence how you will live longer and healthier.

1. Move—find ways to move mindlessly, make moving unavoidable.
2. Know your purpose in life.
3. Down shift – work less, slow down, rest, take a vacation.
4. 80% Rule – stop eating when you're 80% full.
5. Plant-Power – more vegetables, green foods, fruit, less protein and processed foods.
6. Red Wine – for antioxidant benefits – in moderation, however. (NOTE: *There are newer, non-alcoholic sources from the muscadine grape. Resveratrol is a key to several constitutents found in red grapes.* *See page 69, "Resveratrol", for complete information.*)
7. Belong to a social network.
8. Participate and believe in a strong spiritual base.
9. Make family a priority.

These are powerful guidelines. It is through your commitment to your quality of life that you will boost your ability to be successful in losing weight. How you integrate these factors into your life makes a enormous difference in your health and emotional well-being.

TEN ☙ TIPPING THE SCALE ON WEIGHT LOSS

America is the richest nation in the world, with abundant funds available for medical research, specialized health centers and miracle surgical procedures. There are major breakthroughs in the treatment of diseases. However, we are not the healthiest: The World Health Organization ranks the U.S. at 37 when compared to 191 other countries.[81]

Nearly 80% of non-insulin dependent diabetics (NIDDM) are obese. An estimated $11.3 billion dollars are spent annually to diagnose, treat, and manage non-insulin diabetics, which includes treatment for diabetic coma, diabetic eye disease, diabetic ketoacidosis, and diabetic kidney disease.[82]

Obesity accounts for $22.2 billion, or 19 percent, of the total cost of heart disease, including $1.5 million dollars for obesity-related high blood pressure.[83] Treating disease is a profitable business.

While there is growing evidence that Americans and the medical profession have gotten some of the message regarding the connection between what they eat and rate of obesity, there are other complex factors that indicate that there are no simple solutions. People continue to die from obesity-related diseases.

It isn't necessary to elaborate on the hundreds of so-called miracle diet programs that have inundated the marketplace during the past 30 years. This information is readily available on the internet or found in a book store. What is really important is to continue with current scientific research and develop safe weight management programs free of gimmicks, imbalanced processed "diet" foods, and isolated supplements or the promotion of very low caloric intake. Low calorie intake, especially in the elderly, can promote health issues. Programs that are too complicated or severe with needless expenses are not favorable when it comes to having a rewarding experience.

Glycemic Index

It doesn't take but a few minutes to realize that there is an American fixation on food, dieting, and exercise. Many aware individuals have made great stride in modifying their lifestyle and getting healthy. Astonishingly, Americans are still getting fatter by the minute. We continue to examine the reasons behind this concern.

There has been a great deal of information concerning the glycemic index (GI) in several diet programs. The glycemic index ranks carboyhydrates according to their effect on our blood glucose levels after we eat. A very important concept is to understand that not all carbohydrates *behave* in the same way when consumed. For example, Jacobs and Steffen (2003)[84] made a point concerning the relationship of the glycemic index to whole grain flour. The GI depends greatly on the particle size of grain products. There is also a relationship to the amount of phytochemicals (plant chemicals) in the food.

The glycemic index is a guideline, especially for regulating diabetics; however, it is also very imperative that we understand how ALL of what we consume, including its source, content, and level of refining, affects insulin levels in the body.

Dissecting food nutrient by nutrient may not tell the entire story as to how we are to assess foods and their effect. It's like studying the body, cell by cell, losing sight of the relevancy of how healthy cells contribute to the entire body.

We tend to point fingers at individual components, nutrients, foods, and situations ignoring how everything works synergistically Whenever the media announce a new scientific discovery, whether in the realm of a nutrient, a biological chemical component, or new sweetener, consumers go on alert, along with the marketing departments of many food companies. The same holds true with something that is perceived as bad. Information, however, tends to be isolated from the entire story. Data can easily be construed to fit the need of the day or be manipulated to avoid stepping on the toes of one food group or industry. It continues to sway information concerning our health from one idea to the next What we avoid may be the very element that supports our health and our weight. A prime example is fat, which is discussed later in this chapter. What is more relevant is what the WHOLE food does in our body. It is the *synergy* of what we eat, its source, what soil nutrients were available to the growing plant, how it is harvested, processed, and stored. These are just a few factors that contribute to how food affects us biochemically, all making a huge difference.

So as you can see, dear reader, this entire dilemma of maintaining an ideal weight is more complex than anyone can imagine. It requires that we look at the real issues surrounding why we continue to become an obese nation.

When a patient transforms his/her way of thinking to gain a better understanding of the relationshp with food, and commits to a long-term lifestyle change, then the journey to maintaining an ideal weight becomes a permanent change with a greater quality of life extension.

ELEVEN ☙ POWER NUTRIENTS

For the past 20 years, I have continued to research and prescribe a system of weight loss that when followed has produced a 99% success rate among my patients. A good portion of my food recommendations are based on making Lifestyle changes that include healthy eating and exercise habits.

During a 1993 conference in Cambridge, Massachusetts, Oldways (a non-profit research organization that does scientific studies on healthy eating pattterns), and the Harvard School of Public Health concluded that the *Mediterranean Diet* is the "gold standard" for promoting eating patterns that result in life-long good health.[85] Originally created by Aegean (Greek) Islanders, this model is closely tied to the eating traditions derived in the areas of olive oil cultivation in Mediterranean regions. It is rich in fiber, antioxidant polyphenol compounds, vitamins, minerals, and omega-3 fats found in wild fish, grass-fed poulty, and green plants. As a result of the 1993 conference, a new Mediterranean Pyramid was established and it was adapted to several cultural regions working with the foods found in each. In the Lyon Diet Heart Study, a Mediterranean diet supplemented with fish oil capsules showed that the men in the study had substantially reduced mortality and morbidity compared with men in a control diet group.[86], [87] Additionally, it has been endorsed also by the Mayo Clinic.[88]

This healthful pattern delivers equivalent decreases in disease and promotes longevity. I have based a great deal of my program on this model, along with focused consistent motivational counseling during patient visits.

TWELVE ☙ COLOR MY IMMUNITY

A surplus of scientific evidence surrounds the benefits of many substances that are critical for our cell structures, healthy tissue and normal body functions. Director of Human Nutrition at UCLA, David Heber, MD, elaborates on the key elements for maintaining a healthy cell DNA.[89] He categorizes numerous foods and their benefits by their color since they add more diversity into one's diet. Most importantly, they also represent numerous plant chemicals that are beneficial for our immune system to help back up the natural DNA defense systems as we age.

The body is made up of many different cells. Cells divide in a very organized, controlled way when the body requires more. When cells get old or are damaged they are replenished. This is a normal process. If cell DNA becomes damaged, mutations may occur that affects cell growth. When this occurs they don't die when they should and may become erratic causing excess growth that shows up as tumors. [90] A key example of this are the skin growths caused from excessive sun exposure.

There is a prime argument for maintaining a healthy immune system through high intake of plant foods. Heber's studies also found that

- Cancer risks are reduced by 50% in countries that consume a pound of fruits and vegetables every day.[91]
- Substances in fruits and vegetables help maintain a healthy DNA. Eighty to ninety percent of all cancers are a result of a lifetime of accumulated DNA damage and again prevented through increased fruit and vegetable intake.
- Free radical damage increases with age and is reported to be involved with the development of Alzheimer's and other brain disorders.

France, Spain, Switzlerand, Japan tend to have lower heart disease. The CDC reports West Virginia, Kentucky, and Mississippi have the highest rate of heart disease in the U.S. Colorado, the District of Columbia and Hawaii are the lowest.[92] What people eat varies regionally. When you study the reasons, there is a correlation of poverty rates, cultural norms, and education.

Oxidatative stress (free radicals) increases with obesity, leading to more DNA damage that increases health risks (Heber, 2009, p. 8)[93]

A diet high in refined foods, especially refined carboyhydrates, and low on DNA-protecting fruits and vegetables, promotes numerous signals that are sent to our cells, including fat cells. Fat cells release chemicals that encourage inflammation, a key factor in aging and the onset of atherosclerosis, arthritis, heart diease and cancer.

Red/Purple	These foods contain Anthocyanins, powerful anti-oxidants that help cut the risk of heart disease and stroke by inhibiting clot formation. They include blackberries, blueberries, cherries, cranberries, eggplant, plum, prunes, purple or red grapes, raspberries, red apples, red cabbage, red pepper, red wine, strawberries.
Red: Lycopene	A cancer fighting anti-oxidant found in tomatoes and tomato-based food like ketchup or salsa. Lycopene is found in guava, pink grapefruit, and water melon.
Orange	The alpha- beta- carotenes in orange foods boosts eye and skin health and may decrease risk for certain cancers. Acorn or winter squash, apricots, cantaloupe, carrots, mango, pumpkin, sweet potato.
Orange/Yellow	These are rich in beta cryptoxantin, an antioxidant that protects the cells from damage. Nectarines, orange, papaya, peaches, pineapple, tangerines, yellow grapefruit.
Yellow/Green	These foods contain Lutein and Zeaxanthin that protect the eyes from cataracts and macular degeneration. Avocado, collard greens, mustard or turnip greens, corn, cucumbers, green beans, green peas, green or yellow pepper, honeydew, kiwi, romaine or leaf lettuce, spinach, zucchini with skin.

Diversity is a key element in boosting our immune system. It is important for the mind as well. Daily, we must consume a variety of vegetables and fruits in order to give our cells enough nutrient chemicals to maintain a strong immune system. Additionally, activity, both mentally and physically, supports our health. Our immune system is a powerful body organization that keeps us alive. Without this complex mechanism we would quickly die.

THIRTEEN ∞ ACID/ALKALINITY

Ample intake of fruits and vegetables are important for proper pH balance in the body. When the body remains in an acidic state it leads to inflammation and disease.[94] The body is alkaline by design but acid by function, since both components are necessary. Digestion requires alkaline for starches and acid for protein. Medical physiologists and biochemists have indicated that proper pH balance is vital for health. The body however should remain in an alkaline state of pH 7.4 for equilibrium. Diseases such as colds and flu cannot live in alkalinity. Slight chemical variations in body fluids or systems can lead to sickness. Keep in mind that there are some body areas, such as the surface of the skin and the intestines, that remain more acidic to discourage the growth of disease-causing bacteria.

Acidic foods include meats, cheeses, milk coffee, liquor, soda, bread, and artificial sweeteners. They should be balanced with vegetables, fruit and other alkaline foods.

Raw and green organic fruits and vegetables should be high on the shopping list, along with cruciferous fare such as broccoli, cabbage, brussel sprouts, and cauliflower, turnips and kale. Organic meats and poultry and wild fish are good sources of protein. Non-meat protein is also available from soy and vegetables.

FOURTEEN ∞ ANTIOXIDANTS

The three hundred trillion cells in our body require energy to build tissue and organs. Each cell is a miniature factory in itself that contains all the necessary materials to build protein, the building block for all body structures. Inside the cell are mechanisms called organelles that are responsible for the manufacturing of protein. The cell also has its own "energy rooms" called the mitochondria that store oxygen and chemical components made from vitamins and minerals. There can be numerous mitochondria in each cell. When there is a demand for cell energy, it is the task of the mitochondria to convert food chemicals into energy by mixing them with oxygen to produce water and energy. It is a natural metabolic process of every cell and necessary for optimal cellular function.

Free Radicals (Oxidative Stress)

During this oxidation process, reactive free radicals intermediates (ROS – reactive oxygen species) are produced that cause a cascade of chain reactions some of which can be damaging to tissue if not kept in check. Free radicals attack cell DNA, cell membranes, lipids and proteins.

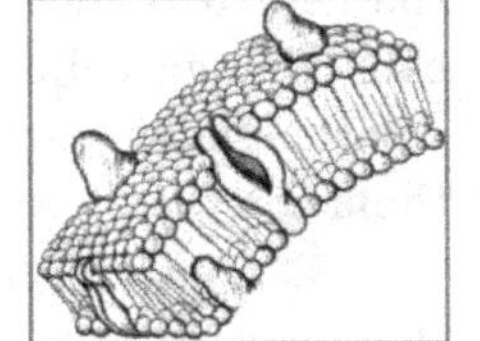

A cell is encased in a lipid bi-layer or plasma membrane that is highly protective for cell contents. Excessive free radicals, also known as unstable molecular species, can destroy this membrane and contribute to tissue breakdown, especially in the collagen networks in body organs, including the skin. A good example of excessive free radical damage is wrinkled skin and premature aging when there is DNA and mitochondrial damage.

Given that we are surrounded by oxygen, we have built- in natural defense systems that help prevent free radical destruction (oxidation). They include complex enzyme systems such as Catalase, superoxide dismutase (SOD) and other peroxidases, and coenzyme **Q10** (Co**Q10**), amino acids such as glutathione (GSH), considered the master intracellular antioxidant. Beta-carotene, vitamins C and E are necessary antioxidants. [95] They help to inhibit and remove free radicals. Antioxidants 'give up' their life in order to neutralize and destroy these interlopers.

Antioxidants are found in the biochemistry of plants as well as in our body. They play a critical role in keeping cells healthy and reduce the affects of what is known as "oxidative stress." Cells can produce oxidative stressors and are capable of detoxifying them during the normal cell function. The arguments for eating high anti-oxidant foods are certainly justified by consuming colorful fresh fruits and vegetables.

Cells are bombarded with a significant number of free radicals and oxidants. Poor diet, excessive sunlight, drugs, radiation, smoking, elevated LDL, low es-trogen deficiency, atherosclerosis, airborne toxins and pollution all contribute to oxidative stress. A full range of antioxidants is required in the cell to reduce an oxidative reactive molecule before they can damage cellular components. They can either prevent intermediate reactive species from being formed or remove them completely.

Diets high in colorful vegetables and fruits bring to the body gifts of exogenous antioxidants that support the immune system. Phytochemicals are also naturally occurring in plants. Substantial research concludes that they are a key component to boosting our immune system in order to prevent disease. They must be present in ample amounts every day. Diversity is very important, and in fact, some state that it is not so much what we eat, but, the diversity in food choices with emphasis on fruits/vegetables – brightly colored foods.

ANTIOXIDANTS

Vitamin C Ascorbic Acid Water soluble	Must be present for the synthesis of collagen that forms the connective tissue; vital for cholesterol regulation, hormone production, detoxification, adrenal synthesis and aides absorption of iron, stimulates immune response. Prevents scurvy.
Vitamin E Lipid Soluble	A group of eight different but related fat soluble vitamins. Alpha-tocopherol has the highest bioavailability and is well metabolized by the body. Protects cell membranes and the skin. It mitigates lipid radicals produced in the lipid peroxidation chain reaction.
Vitamin A Lipid Soluble	Complex of fat soluble molecules called carotenoids – beta-carotene and lycopene. Beta Carotene is a precursor to vitamin A
Phytochemicals	Found naturally in plants. Polyphenols are most powerful and contain numerous anti-inflammatory properties. The include • Resveratrol (phenolic compound) • Ellagic Acid • Proanthocyanidins • Bioflavanoids • Stilbenes • Polyphenolics • Anthocyanins[96] • Stilbenes

Resveratrol

For years, red wine has been an integral part of the diets of the French and the Mediterranean people. They have less heart disease due to their diet, which includes consumption of red wine. The polyphenols in red wine appear to have great protective properties. [97] In particular is the resveratrol with its anti-inflammatory and high anti-oxidant properties. It has been found to have positive cardiovascular and anti-cancer effects. Much of resveratrol is found in the skin of red grapes where it serves as a natural antibiotic for the grape that helps it to defend itself preventing fungus, heat, humidity, insects and fungi (Hartle, et al, 2008, p. 4). They have been found to protect the heart and brain from oxidized fat, an important factor in the prevention of Alzheimer's. It helps to protect blood vessels and prevent damage caused from free-radicals (Hartle, et al, 2008, pp.5-11).

A 2003 landmark study at Harvard University and the National Institute on Aging found that resveratrol offsets the bad effects of a high-calorie diet in mice and expanded their lifespan.[98] Resveratrol also reversed nearly all of the changes in gene expression patterns found in mice on high calories diets --- some of which are associated with diabetes, heart disease and other diseases related obesity.

Drinking red wine, however, should be done in moderation and it recommended that men consume no more than two glasses a day and women, one. Wine should be consumed during a meal that includes lots of vegetables.

A great non-alcoholic source of resveratrol is found in red grapes. Research has shown that the Muscadine grape contains the high levels of phytochemicals such as ellagic acid, which add large health benefits. Ellagic acid compounds are absent in other grapes (Hartle, et al, 2008, p. 5)

Muscadines are a hardy grape, since they thrive under weather conditions that would normally kill a European variety. Muscadines have an extra pair of chromosomes, which are a contributing factor in their survival rate in the high heat and humidity of the southeastern part of the United States (Hartle, et al, 2008, p. 4-5). They are native to the U.S. and are filled with high levels of phytochemicals that are considered medicinal. The phytonutrients in muscadines have been studied for their effect on metabolic syndrome and aging.

Ph.D scientists, Hartle, Greenspan, and Hargrove conducted Eight years of extensive research in the Nu-traceutical Research Laboratory at the University of Georgia.[99] Muscadine grapes are considered to have the highest level of antioxidant activity than any other grape on the market. Over 397 published papers substantiate the research on resveratrol.[100]

FIFTEEN ☙ ENZYMES

Enzymes are energized protein molecules found in all living cells. They are the catalysts for every chemical process in the body and are essentially necessary for life. Their activity depends upon the presence of vitamins and minerals (copper, iron, calcium or zinc).

Enzymes have been labeled "workers" since they carry out these important tasks such as breaking down fats, carbohydrates and fiber. To maintain a healthy body you require both enzymes and building materials which are the proteins, minerals, and vitamins that would be useless without the presence of enzymes to break them down. Many enzymes are produced in the liver, pancreas, gallbladder and other organs.[101]

There are three types of enzymes, metabolic, digestive, and plant. The largest classification is the metabolic enzymes that play a large role in breathing, talking, moving, thinking, behavior and maintenance of the immune system. They speed up the chemical reaction within the cells for detoxification and energy production. A subset of these enzymes helps to neutralize poisons and carcinogens. Most of the metabolic enzymes are developed in the pancreas.

There are numerous enzymes within the body with multiple functions, including food metabolism/breakdown. They are secreted along the digestive tract, beginning in the mouth. They break food down into nutrients and wastes. Nutrients are then absorbed into the blood stream while wastes are discarded.

Food enzymes enter our body through eating raw foods. Raw food initiates the process of digestion in the mouth and upper stomach. They include proteases for digesting protein, lipases for digesting fats and amylases for digesting carbohydrates. Plant foods bring with them their own supply of enzymes to aid in their digestion. Cooking and processing them destroys them.

The absence of raw foods in the diet places a strain on the pancreas. It becomes over stimulated and depletes a great amount of its enzyme potential by the exaggerated discharge of its secretions.

Cellulose enzymes from plant fibers are also present in raw foods. These beneficial components carry nutrients through the gut wall and transport metal and toxins out.

Raw food enzymes are very compatible with the low acidic pH of the stomach. Pancreatic enzymes are compatible with the alkaline pH of the small intestine and thus we require both sources of enzymes.

The field of enzymes certainly is not a complete field. We can find earlier data, however, pioneered by researchers years ago; in particular, Dr. John Beard (1907) a Scottish embryologist and author of the book *Enzymatic Treatment of Cancer*[102], claimed that most degenerative diseases begin in the digestive system. According to his research, consumption of excess animal protein overworks the pancreas to the point that it malfunctions. It appears that this undigested protein may lead to a toxic fermentation in the intestinal tract leading to symptoms of bloating, gas, abdominal pain and eventual colon irritation.

The pancreas secretes specific enzymes — trypsin and chymotrypsin — that suppress the excessive growth of cells known as trophoblast cells. Trophoblast cells are present for the development of the pancreas. During pancreatic malfunction, however, these cells may become potentially cancerous.

You can easily surmise the reasons why it is so necessary to include large amounts of fruits and vegetables in your diet and to reduce over consumption of meats. Plant based enzymes are beneficial in developing a suitable digestive system and allow the body to produce more metabolic enzymes by reducing the need to produce digestive enzymes. Enzyme activity also mitigates with age, and thus a balanced diet is important throughout our entire life.

SIXTEEN ☙ PROBIOTICS

A healthy digestive and immune system requires a synergistic blend of millions of microorganisms. Residing in the small and large intestine, there are at least 400-500 different varieties of microorganisms.[103] They make up about two pounds of your body weight. Most are hard at work producing a variety of substances that can prevent cancerous tumors, produce natural antibodies, reduce cholesterol, deactivate viruses, and enhance the immune system.[104]

Probiotics essentially are necessary for the proper functioning of all body systems. Most of these intestinal bacteria do not affect our health and live harmoniously performing their duties.

The consumption of carbonated drinks, laxatives, birth control, coffee, alcohol, aging, antacids, stress and antibiotics cause an imbalance in the natural flora and end up contributing to their destruction.[105] This imbalance fosters undesirable bacteria to rapidly increase in numbers. This may lead to illness and long-term health problems due to the toxic compounds they create.

Overuse of broad-spectrum antibiotics has become a health concern and been shown to be detrimental to the natural intestinal flora. There is also growing concern regarding the routine use of antibiotics in domestic animal feed additives, as well as the use of prescription antibiotics.[106] They tend to foster an increase in the growth of unfavorable microorganisms in our body.

The widespread use of low-dose topical anti-bacterial products found in household cleaners, hand soaps, and other lotions may be contributing to drug resistant bacteria. Reports from health agencies confirm that use of these products can be harmful to babies and children.[107]

There is also an alarming 15% increase in pediatric antibiotics since **1990** mostly in the treatment of childhood diseases.[108] That means that up to **50** percent of children in the United States take antibiotics for ear infections three or more times before they reach the age of five.[109]

Again, the typical Western diet — low in dietary fiber, high in meat, high in total fat and high in animal fat and protein — is associated with reduced populations of beneficial microflora that includes Lactobacilli and Bifidobacteria.[110] There is a direct correlation between the reduction of risk factors for cancer with populations who regularly eat probiotic foods such as yogurt and other fermented dairy products.[111]

Probiotics have the ability to prevent the formation of carcinogens in the colon. For example, if bile acids pass into the colon into a field of unhealthy bacteria, they can be quickly transformed into cancer cells. The presence of healthy probiotics quickly opposes and eradicates this process. They also produce short-chain fatty acids — butyric acid — that help regulate normal colon cell growth and death. Butyric acid absorbs and metabolizes potentially carcinogenic chemicals.[112]

Several studies have indicated that there are large benefits to consuming probiotics for the management of or prevention of certain diseases such as peptic ulcers, irritable bowel syndrome (IBS) as well as diarrhea.[113,114]

Sources of probiotics include supplements, live-culture yogurt, some cottage cheeses, kefir, and sweet acidophilus milk.

SEVENTEEN ☙ FATS

Almost thirty years ago we thought we had found the perfect way to lose weight. Fat-free was IN. During the 1980's through public demand, the food industry rose to the occasion and lowered or eliminated fats in many of our foods by 15 percent or more.[115] Food industry research kitchens were busy developing and testing foods that were both lower in carbohydrates and fat. In order to produce a fat-free muffin that has great texture and taste, a recipe high in sugar and other refined ingredients is required to make it taste good. There were over one thousand different fat-free foods developed as a result of consumer demand.[116]

Low fat, low carbohydrates became synonymous with being healthy. Not surprising, these untruths helped us to become the fattest country in the world. We are currently 30% - 40% higher than in the early 1980s.

Basically, we were all ignorant of the real story and the mistakes surrounding the delicate relationship between Lifestyle, body health, and balancing what we ate. We have been programmed to fail through years of flawed dietary advice. Food regimens recommended by many well-meaning authors, national agencies, medical professionals and a multitude of other experts missed the point.

What's even more daunting is that our eating habits cause dangerous biochemical effects that actually can kill us.

Most premature deaths essentially occur due to overweight and the health issues associated with them, specifically an epidemic level of metabolic syndrome.[117] Metabolic syndrome consists of obesity, abnormal levels of cholesterol and triglycerides, high blood pressure, elevated fasting insulin levels, and a predisposition to blood clotting. HOW we eat will make a difference in reducing risk factors.

The Good, the Bad, and the Ugly

We don't' have to give up our love of food to be healthy. The truth about fats is that we require them just as we need protein and carbohydrates. How fats affect us depends upon the type of fat and its source.[118] There are several types of fats that are referred to as saturated and unsaturated. Understand that eating the right kind of fat is essential to longevity. Good fats can actually reduce levels of bad cholesterol and dangerous triglycerides.[119] They also support the resiliency of our cells since they are part of the makeup of a cell membrane. So what exactly are fats?

Fats and oils are made up of carbon molecules framed with hydrogen and oxygen molecules. When a carbon chain is completely full of hydrogen molecules it is considered "saturated". When it is missing two hydrogen molecules, it is called a monosaturated fat (Vigilante, 1999, pp. 45-52).[120]

Monosaturated fats Sources	**Appearance**: Solid at room temperature. **Source**: Shortening, butter, lard, shortening, meat fat. **Risk Factor**: inflammation, heart disease, increased blood pressure, stroke diabetes, gallbladder issues, breast cancer, ovarian cancer **Recommendation**: Limit
Trans fats – Polyunsaturated fats Hydrogenation	**Appearance:** Liquid **Sources**: vegetable oils - corn oil, saf-flower, canola. If cold pressed and unprocessed they may have health benefits. Unfortunately they become trans fatty acids by chemically adding hydrogen to prevent oxidation and extend the shelf life. They become very dangerous to cells and our health since they do not occur naturally in nature. They decrease insulin sensitivity by making the cell membrane stiff and inflexible. **Recommendation:** Avoid
Liquid monounsaturated	**Sources:** Olives, olive oil, and limited in nuts and avocadoes **Benefits**: Olive oil contains anti-inflammatory properties
Essential Fatty Acids Omega 3 (DHA, ALA, EPA) Omega 6 (linoleic acid (LA) makes arachidonic acid (AA) Omega-3 must be consumed in a ratio of 3:2-4	Building blocks of fats and oils are called fatty acids. Essential fatty acids are fats that we don't manufacture in our body. We must obtain from food with regular intake. **Benefits**: Cardiovascular - Reduces blood pressure; lowers risk of colon, breast, prostate cancers; anti-inflammatory (arthritis); psoriasis, anti-free radical, ADD & ADHD, reduces stress chemicals cortisol, norepinephrine; helps with depression, improves mood, mental clarity. **Source**: sockeye salmon, borage, evening primrose

The Good Fat

Omega fatty acids (Essential Fatty Acids or EFAs) are essential for health and they must be present for wound healing and for all cell membranes. They are not manufactured by our body so we must obtain them from our food. When we consume vegetables, white meats, grains, seeds, beef, pork, and lamb, we receive ample amount of Omega-6s. On the other hand, we do not always consume ample amount of Omega-3s.

Essential fatty acids contain essential ingredients from which many body hormones are manufactured.[121] Deficiency in essential fatty acids results in dehydration, skin aging, sterility in men, miscarriages in women, arthritis and inflammation, poor tissue oxygenation, loss of collagen, wrinkles, skin pigmentation, distended capillaries and diffuse redness.[122] They are also a key for anti-aging.

During a five year breakthrough study, University of California researcher, Farzaneh-Far and his colleagues found that heart patients on higher omega-3 levels experienced a lower rate of decay in their chromosomes' protective caps (telomeres).[123] This anti-aging effect is attributed to omega-3s documented antioxidant effects and their ability to stimulate production of an enzyme that repairs the telomeres.[124]

An important feature of omega acids is that they are essential to healthy cell membranes and proper function of nerve cells in the brain. Omega-3s are required by the brain cells and their long nerves to manufacture insulated membranes that need to be impermeable and prevent interference to the rate and flow of neurotransmission.[125] Research has found that when babies are nursed they have optimum brain growth and development.[126], [127] It is important that nursing mothers consume adequate amounts of these vital essential fatty acids.

Studies with ADD and ADHD children show that they lack essential fatty acids in their body. Remedial nutritional therapy that includes essential fatty acids may help improve this condition. In his latest book, *The NDD Book*, William Sears, MD explores through case studies the significance of nutrition and how it affects the brains and behavior of children. When there were significant changes to their diet, there was major improvement in learning and behavior.[128]

Omega-3's (DHA) and Omega-6's (DHA) improve cell sensitivity to insulin. However, the ratio of Omegas 3 should be in a ratio of 3:6.[129], [130] As we age, cells become resistant to the effects of insulin, which can result in the increase of body fat. Insulin resistance occurs with individuals that have elevated levels of blood fats, heart disease and Type 2 diabetes.

I cannot speak enough about the value of essential fatty acids in the diet, especially omega-3. It is important to consume omega-3 and omega-6 in the correct ratio. If you live in the U.S., it is not necessary to supplement with mega-6, since most people obtain an abundance of omega-6s from cooking oils, meats, poultry and other prepared foods. The American Heart Association recommends a daily intake of 1-4 grams a day of Omega-3, depending upon your health. If you are required to lower triglycerides, it is recommended to take 2 to 4 grams of EPA+DHA daily.[131] Always check with your doctor if you are on medications.

Consider the source carefully, especially when pregnant. Avoid farm raised fish and fish that may have high levels of contaminants. Purchase wild caught salmon from cold waters that are from sustainable fisheries such as in cold Alaskan waters.[132], [133] It will keep your skin healthy, as well as every cell in your body.

Olive Oil

Olive oil has been a dietary food for centuries in the Mediterranean part of the world, where Greeks and Italians experience little heart disease. It has a large amount of unsaturated fatty acids and a high content of antioxidants. Olive oil contains a very small amount of essential fatty acids; however, it has about 75 percent of a nonessential monounsaturated fatty acid called oleic acid. It plays a very important role in supporting the transport of omega-3s into the cell membranes.

The benefits of olive oil are far-reaching, with substantial research that backs up its claims. Virgin olive oil (must be cold pressed) have been found to lower blood pressure, decrease the stickiness of platelets and protect from heart attacks.[134] It also is protective to the stomach helping to prevent stomach ulcers. Oleic acid decreases oxidation of LDLs (bad cholesterols) and helps prevent the buildup of arterial plaque. Other benefits[135], [136]

- Decreases LDL cholesterol
- Increases HDL cholesterol
- Supports intestinal absorption of nutrients
- Lowers blood pressure
- Oxidative stress
- Stimulates pancreatic secretions
- Prevents osteoporosis
- Helps lower glucose levels in diabetics
- Reduces risk of prostate, breast, and colon cancers
- Prevents edema (water retention)
- Supports the gall bladder activity

Not all olive oils are alike. When purchasing olive oil consider the source. Read labels carefully because some olive oils are mixed with canola oil. Cold pressed virgin oils produced in the Mediterranean area of the world are considered the best since they contain high contents of a component called hydroxytyrosol.[137]

- **Extra virgin** - considered the best, least processed, comprising the oil from the first pressing of the olives. Contains the highest level of antioxidants and vitamin E and phenols since it is less processed.
- **Virgin** - from the second pressing.
- **Pure** - undergoes some processing, such as filtering and refining.
- **Extra light** - undergoes considerable processing and only retains a very mild olive flavor.

Store all olive oil in a dark place and do not expose to excessive light since it causes it to oxidize.

Coconut Oil

Growing up in Manila, we used coconut oil in our diet. Coconut oil is a saturated fat that has medium chained fatty acids and monoglycerides found to have great benefits. It contains lauric acid and capric acid, which convert to monolaurin in the body. Monolaurin is an antibacterial, anti-viral and antiprotozoal substance that is used by human body to destroy lipid-coated viruses such as HIV, herpes, influenza, various pathogenic bacteria and protozoa such as *Giardia lamblia* — an intestinal parasite.[138]

During the 1980s and based on earlier statements in the late 1950s, it received some abusive rhetoric stating that coconut oil along with all saturated oils were causing heart issues. This statement, made by some special interest groups, was totally false since the real perpetrator of heart disease was the hydrogenation of oils to give them longer shelf life. The trans-fat danger has finally gained recognition — they are the culprit.

Coconut oil may be used in cooking and sautéing since it is stable oil and does not turn into trans-fats through heat. It is important that it is obtained from a reliable organic source.

EIGHTEEN ☙ WATER — BEVERAGE FOR LIFE

Daily consumption of fresh, pure water is vital to human survival. The human body is about 75 percent water, with 25 percent solid matter. Each cell is made up of about 75% water. Your blood is 82 percent water. The brain is 70% water since it is bathed in cerebrospinal fluid. Water is necessary for digestion, elimination of food wastes in the body, and regulating body temperature.[139] Peak performance during sports workouts requires water. Dehydration in as much as 2 percent can decrease athletic performance.[140]

Individual requirements will vary from person to person. For some people, 8 glasses a day will be enough, while for others, it may be more or less.[141]

So how do you determine if you are hydrated? You can easily get an idea of your body hydration levels by the color of your urine. If it is clear with almost no color, this may be a good indicator that you are well-hydrated. The darker it is, the more dehydrated you are.

Dehydration causes loss of bodily functions and can produce damage to the body. Many individuals, especially in older age, develop dehydration conditions simply because they lose their sense of thirst. Consequently, there is a reduction in daily water intake.[142] Coffee, tea, soda, and other similar drinks do add liquid into the body; however, they are not a substitute for pure water.

Choose your water source carefully. Most tap water is filled with chlorine and other contaminants.[143] Additionally, bottled water has come under question. A four-year study of 103 brands of bottled water done by the Natural Resources Defense Council found that one-third contained levels of bacteria or carcinogens that exceeded purity guidelines.[144] There are newer home water-filtering devices that will improve the quality of your water without destroying minerals.

The Gift of Water

- When on a weight loss program, water assists in transporting fats and eliminates toxic waste products.
- Prevents clogging of arteries in the heart and brain.
- Helps to relieve headaches and hangovers
- Helps reduce constipation.
- Helps relieve heartburn.
- Relieves muscle aches.
- Increases the efficiency of the immune system.
- Helps the body to replenish its supply of the neurotransmitter serotonin during times of depression.
- Required for the production of melatonin, natures sleep regulator.
- Generates electrical and magnetic impulses in all cells.
- Aids in strong bone formation helping to prevent osteoporosis.
- Normalizes the blood-manufacturing systems that aid in cancer prevention.
- Necessary for brain function where it energizes brain cells.

Dehydration

Dehydration encourages aging and inflammation. There is research indicating that many root causes of disease is dehydration.[145] It is vital that we consume water BEFORE we feel thirst. Individuals with asthma, allergies and heartburn should maintain a state of hydration at all times.

Aging and the Importance of Water

Regulation of water in the body can be referred to as the body's drought- and resource-management program (Batamanghelidj, 2003, p. 55).[146] Water is the central regulator of energy and osmotic balance in the body. There are electrical energy generating properties of water that help convert food into energy, as well as regulate other cellular functions. When you drink a glass of water, it makes its way into your cells where its molecules become highly organized in order to meet the polarity requirements of the thousands of chemical reactions necessary for cell function. This intracellular water molecularly adapts to individual cell functions to support protein structures and other metabolic processes (Batamanghelidj. 2003, pp. 26-27).[147]

The ability for optimum water regulation in the body mitigates with age reducing cell efficiency. It is important that elderly people maintain good hydration levels. So how else can we replenish and maintain the hydration levels of our body cells?

Eating raw vegetables and fresh fruit juices is an ideal way to obtain water that is readily utilized by the body. Eating juicy fruits like water melon, honeydew, apples, and grapes contain valuable enzymes, vitamins, and fiber.

Water and Stress

During times of chronic stress, the body goes into a fight-or-flight mode. There is a physiological change in the body, including dilated pupils, increased heart rate, release of glucose and fatty acids and other chemical changes such as adrenal overload that all cascade into a change of body fluids. Too much stress places the body into a state of severe dehydration, thereby forcing the body to ration its water reserves. The body is very selective and provides it where it is needed the most. The brain is the first area to ration water over all other systems (Batmanghelidj, 2003, pp. 122-123).[148] Persistent dehydration continues to affect other body systems eventually leading to breakdown.

Drugs are powerful for controlling and warding off harmful bacteria and regulating certain condition. Drugs may also mask the real reason behind an illness. Many illnesses may be reduced just by increasing water intake and changing dietary programs.

Water is the elixir of life; without it, life cannot exist. No other liquid can sustain digestion and overall health and well-being.

NINETEEN ☙ THE AIR THAT WE BREATHE

Breathing is a requisite of life and we cannot live very long without air. An average adult breathes about 20 cubic meters or 20,000 liters of air a day.[149] The quality of life depends upon effective breathing, taking in enough oxygen for the blood stream and then removal of carbon dioxide. An individual's ability to breathe clean, pure air directly affects his or her quality of life and health.

Air is made up of elements such as oxygen, carbon, and nitrogen and combinations of element, called compounds. Minute particles of dust and dirt are also present in air. Elements and compounds make up the air we breath and they must be in balance. When imbalanced, they become pollutants that affect air quality.

Pollution can make both people and animals sick. Too much pollution can destroy the paint on our cars and interfere with our own intake of oxygen. Pollutants vary, depending upon geographical location. The most common pollutants include:

- Particulate Matter (smoke, soot, dirt) all coming from factories, or from cars traveling over dry roads.
- Sulphur dioxide (SO2): combinations of sulfur and oxygen atoms called sulfur oxide can be harmful to vegetation including agricultural crops. When combined with ammonia it forms very fine particle matter. When mixed with moisture it becomes acid rain. Acid rain is harmful to humans, animals and vegetation and discolors or damages buildings.
- Nitrogen Dioxide and Oxides (NO2, NOx): When nitrogen oxide mixes with oxygen it becomes NO2 and appears yellowish or brownish depending on the density. Nitrogen oxides form when fossil fuels are burned in motor vehicles, trains, airplanes, power plants, heating devices and factories.
- Carbon monoxide: Carbon monoxide is produced by burning fossil fuels such as gasoline, diesel, natural gas, fuel oil, or coal. Cars are a major source of carbon monoxide in the air. Wood burning, agricultural burning, industrial combustion and forest fires also produce carbon monoxide.

It is important to maintain good air quality that is clean and free from bacteria and other forms of molds and other air borne inflictions.

Since the energy crisis of the 1970s, our homes have more insulation, tighter windows and doors and do not "breathe" the way they did years ago. We do not always open windows to air out our homes and offices. In warmer climates, air conditioning may be operated to cool buildings. This closed environment harbors mold and other bacteria, hiding dangers right inside the walls or ductwork. It is not uncommon for people to spend 8-16 hours indoors without ever going outside. Unhealthy environments and poor ventilation can result in poor productivity and the spread of illnesses.

Eighty percent of flus and viruses are caused by contact with germs on surfaces. It is important that individuals frequently wash their hands, especially when in public places like schools and hospitals.

If we are going to spend most of our time in a closed environment, then it is important to have quality indoor air. There is now newer, university-tested technology for air purification systems that destroy airborne and surface microbes.

TWENTY ☙ THE BIGGER PICTURE

In any weight loss program WHAT we choose to eat and HOW we live impacts our daily well-being. It is also important that we discuss the importance of maintaining a strong immune system, beginning with a conscious effort to examine our overall Lifestyle and commitment to optimum health.

Worthy of mention is that our quality of health now hangs in a sea of new compromise, being greatly impaired by increased exposure to inappropriate antibiotic usage during the past **40-50** years The outcome is the creation of antibiotic-resistent *superbugs.*

- Methicillin-resistant staphylococcus aureus (MRSA)
- Clostridium difficile (C. Diff)
- Vancomycin-resistant enterococci (VRE)

Interestingly enough, these organisms are natural in the environment without making healthy people sick.[150]

Staphylococcus aureus is natural to our body and has been around since the **1960**s. It colonizes on the skin and in the nasal passages of approximately **30**% of Americans. Approximately 1% of people are now colonized with a mutated form of *Staph aureus* that is an antibiotic-resistant superbug called MRSA. It is resistant to penicillin and other drugs and causes extreme illness, even death. Individuals who enter a hospital for a minor injury could end up dying from MRSA if contracted. MRSA is relentless in its attack to those who may have a weakened immune system.[151]

Clostridium difficile (C. Diff) lives all around us and in our digestive system. Normally, it doesn't cause problems until an individual takes antibiotics for another reason. *C. Diff* can colonize out of control, making an individual even sicker.

There are presently over **500,000** reported cases of infection in the U.S. Ninety-nine thousand die each year from these hospital-acquired infections.

What has happened to the American body during the past 35 years has lead to a pandemic of obesity including the diseases that originate from a compromised immune system. We have grown into a nation of sensationalism, false pretenses and platitudes, losing sight of what is really important in helping us to become productive, vital human beings that live in essential health.

Dr. O's Lifestyle Changes for Enhanced Health formula:

Nutrition + Water + Air + Exercise & Activity + Adequate Rest + Positive Mental Attitude = Wellness, Health Maintenance, Weight Reduction and Balance

ঌ৪ঌ

IV

MIND – BODY WEIGHT LOSS

"Weight loss involves much more than counting calories and eating the right foods. Losing weight is not about the body – it's about the mind. It's about changing the way you think about food. It's also about changing the way you think about life. Your weight is the most visible reflection of who you are and losing weight involves nothing short of fundamentally changing your life. Change your life first and the weight will come off naturally – and stay off."

The RAVE Diet & Lifestyle
by Mike Anderson

ONE ꟈ POWER OF THE MIND

"Our human software runs in the forefront of our minds, telling us where we can go, with whom we can go, and what is possible for us when we get there. Most of us will never know ourselves outside the confines of this automatic conditioning. We will never know what's possible beyond our current belief systems constructed by our shame and fear. These messages are deeply encoded in our psyches."[152]

Debbie Ford - *Why Good People Do Bad Things*

Change your thoughts — change your life!

At the dawn of each day in our modern life appear consistent reminders that we have within us the power to choose and alter our thoughts and reactions. What greatly influences this ability is our *knowledge, awareness* and *consciousness.* There is little excuse for the contrary given that we exist in an age of information with reams of data flowing through cyberspace, television, and books and other print media. How attentive we are, and what moves us through patterns of being stuck-in-the-box, is determined through our *willingness* and *desire* to alter our present beliefs and look at life though a cascade of sheer possibility.

What sways this ability, are our thoughts and reactions that literally affect millions of communication signals permeating throughout our 300 trillion body cells. At any given microsecond with an infinitesimal shift of a thought, life as we know it can quickly be altered to our demise OR become something greater than our thoughts and belief systems that transform into absolute joy and happiness. Given that we are dealing with human nature, this is not as easy as it sounds. It takes some work.

So what does all of this mind matter have to do with weight loss? Anderson's quote is relevant. *Weight loss involves much more than counting calories and eating the right foods. Losing weight is not about the body – it's about the mind. It's about changing the way you think about life.* [153], [154]

The Ultimate Tune-up

Prior to embarking on a weight loss program, I advise you to closely examine your present thoughts (subconscious and conscious) as well as how you currently view your body. Second, it is recommended to engage in a total inventory of your life — physically and emotionally, including your environment and lifestyle. Stop and take the time to give your life a tune-up.

Change your thoughts, change your biology. There is a multifaceted mind/body connection to our failures and successes in life. Understanding this connection is a key to being mindful as to why we go "on and off" diets and why we gain weight.

Survival and health are determined through biological networks that are responsible for communicating and regulating body functions throughout complex groups of cells, organs, and systems. A highly synchronized process, cells respond to millions of biochemical signals influenced by their natural environment. These cues move along pathways that help regulate cellular activities and influence cell behavior. What ultimately directs the synchronicity and success of this process are our thoughts and emotions, that influence both the *quality* and outcome of this process.[155] So how does this happen?

Mind Power

There are two distinct and separate subdivisions of the mind, the *conscious* and the *subconscious.*[156] The subconscious mind is a warehouse of stimulus tapes, such as those that are responsible for instinctive behavior (fight or flight) and learned behavior (our habits). Conversely, the *conscious* mind is responsible for our creativity and conscious thoughts. An important piece of information is to realize that many of our subconscious beliefs influence our behavior. For example, when we were six years old we were told that we couldn't leave the table until we ate everything on our plate. That earlier message influenced that it was important that we eat until our plate is empty. Fast forward to 45. We are still compelled to eat everything on our plate.

The prefrontal cortex in the front of our brain is associated with thinking, planning, and decision-making. Scientists indicate that this is the seat of the *self-conscious* or the place where we process information for an immediate decision (reaction).[157] It has access to data in our long-term memory bank (our history) that allows us to compile information that affects our daily decisions. In other words, we have the ability to *self-reflect.* The self-conscious can observe our behavior, evaluate it, and make a conscious decision to change the program. Accordingly, the self-conscious mind is very powerful. In other words, we have the power to choose how to respond to any environmental signal — the experiences — past and present — that cause us to react. We have the power to say yes or no.

Healthy weight loss begins with having a healthy brain.[158] It is not just will power alone or lack of desire. A quick fix isn't always the answer either as observed in patients having gastric banding. Ten years post procedure shows that the success rate is approximately 31 percent.[159]

Research presented at the 2009 Society of Ingestive Behavior annual meeting found that depressed patients who followed a six-month behavioral weight-loss program lost weight reported a significant drop in their symptoms of depression.[160] Healthy life style means a happier life.

TWO ☙ THE BUCK STOPS HERE.... OR DOES IT? THE DNA CONNECTION

So again, what does all this cell matter have to do with losing weight?

Studies on the role of DNA in cells have been performed since the late 1940s. Remarkable findings from scientists delving deep into the workings of a single cell — especially the nucleus and cell membrane — revealed some very elating data.

At one point in time the nucleus was believed to be the *brain* of the cell. The question was to determine how important it was to a cell function and whether it was possible for the cell to maintain normal functioning if it was removed.[161]

Biologists developed a small microscopic pipette and passed it into the cytoplasm of a cell and carefully withdrew the nucleus. The cell actually recovered and continued to live and carry on cellular activity, including building protein and communicating with other cells. This discovery was important since it resulted in the realization that cells are influenced by more than just the nucleus. A key function, however, of the nucleus is that it contains chromosomal contents of DNA, including regulatory proteins, that direct the *rebuilding* of the cell and its parts during the normal physiological processes of daily activity.[162,163] While cells can exist without their nucleus for a short period of time, removing the ability for repair or cell division eventually results in cell death.[164] It's like taking away the control tower and repair managers at an airport— the planes can land for a while due to the ability of the pilots who know how to fly and land airplanes and possess a basic understanding of maintenance. Sooner or later, however, directional and maintenance resources become exhausted, and it leads to operation dysfunction and final shutdown.

Genetic Destiny

So aren't we all a product of our genetics?

Dr. B.H. Lipton[165] explains that there are two mechanisms by which organisms pass on hereditary information. The first involves what is naturally inherited — the blueprints responsible for directing our initial development and cell regeneration and processes.

The second is the alteration that occurs in these genes as a result of our external environmental experiences. This can also influence what is passed from one generation to the next. This is a powerful finding. Beginning in the womb, experiences of adverse nutritional and environmental circumstances throughout fetal and neonatal periods of development can greatly affect the future health of the child. [166,167] In contrast, it has also been shown that an enriched environment can override genetic mutations. Our attitude, lifestyle and responses affect the future quality of our own life as well as that of our children.

Past conventional thought for genetic determinism stated that cellular blueprints — the DNA — were solely responsible for our mind/body development, including our beliefs and inevitable fate in life. For example, it was believed that our DNA determined how we would age, how many wrinkles we would get, and whether or not we would grow to an old age. Moreover, it would lead to the inevitability that we will acquire the arthritis or Alzheimer's that incapacitated our parents or grandparents. We blame genetics on psychological and physiological tendencies and traits such as ADD, depression, alcoholism, addictive behavior, and obesity.

What's more amazing is that we're guided to believe it as absolute truth when we're told that we have six months to live or have an *incurable* disease such as cancer or heart disease. In the end we thought that we had no choice but to surrender to these depilating circumstances and conditions. The prognosis becomes our destiny.

Epigenetics

And now let's look at another possibility. It's THE GOOD NEWS that is found in the fine print in the back of the news room. This should become the headline of our thoughts and realizations that guides us into a healthy future.

Thanks to a modern science called *Epigenetics,* which means "control above genetics," we now recognize that our DNA in fact plays a smaller part; actually 35% is what we've inherited.[168] The other 65% is in our hands to take control and/or take charge of our destiny, especially our health.

According to many scientists, epigenetics is the *new science of self-empowerment.*[169] It is through the event of environmental signaling that arouses a regulatory protein that directs information to the DNA, RNA and the final outcome of new protein and health of a cell.[170],[171]

Our survival and our health are related to the efficiency of good signal transfer. Clinical studies led by founder Doe Childre, and his researchers at the Institute of HeartMath in Boulder Creek, California have confirmed that "measureable molecular changes in the DNA molecule can result from human desire, intentions, and emotions."[172],[173] A new paradigm shift has emerged in the field of genetic studies as a result of the findings of these scientists.

During the 1970s, researcher Candace Pert, Ph.D., *Molecules of Emotion*, established a bio-molecular basis for our emotions through her dynamic discovery of the opiate receptor and other peptide receptors in the brain and the body.[174] Her research scientifically established that our internal chemicals, the neuropeptides and their receptors were actually the biological foundations of our awareness — emotions, beliefs and expectations. They influence how we respond to daily occurrences and ultimately our ability to function in the world. Pert's research also illustrated that the *mind* is not just in the brain. It is in every cell found in a complex communication network throughout the entire body.

Mind-Body Media

Towards the end of the 20th Century, there was a deluge of interest impelled by some medical doctors, researchers and other enlightened individuals around the globe. During 1993, a groundbreaking PBS series and later book, *Healing and The Mind*, acclaimed author and television journalist, Bill Moyers, interviewed world-renowned experts in the field of the mind-body connection and medicine.[175]

Among those experts was David Eisenberg, who spent 11 years in China studying traditional Chinese medicine (TCM) where Western and Chinese medicine exist together. The positive benefits of massage were also included in his studies. Eisenberg's work includes the integration of medical practices of TCM into Western medicine for the improvement of health and healing.

Margaret Kemeny, Ph.D., a psychologist with postgraduate training in immunology and psycho-neuroimminology discussed her research with emotions and its relationship to the immune system. Her studies included the relationship of the immune response with both stressful (fight or flight) and elated experiences. In the initial stage of an emotion of fear, the body's immune cells experienced a positive increase. When an individual's experience of fear is prolonged over a period of time, however, the immune system no longer responds positively and begins to run the risk of ending up with physiological responses that are no longer adaptive.[176] Additional study of depression states leads to biological changes that make the body more vulnerable to heart attacks and other maladies. [177]

THREE ☙ FOOD AND CELL HEALTH

During the 1950s, Nobel Prize winner and Danish scientist, Jens Christian Skou discovered unique pumping systems (sodium/potassium pumps) found within cell membranes that are responsible for transporting food/wastes in and out of the cells. A process known as *polarization* (a cell's resting stage) and *depolarization* (cellular activity) was further explored by German scientists, Erwin Neher and Bert Sakmann during the 1980s. They were awarded a Nobel Prize for their discoveries involving the function of single ion channels in cells. They were able to insert a glass pipette through a cell, affirming the importance of the cellular membrane in a single cell and total body. What these scientists confirmed is that the electrical polarization/depolarization of cellular membranes is so important for life that approximately *80% of the energy produced from food is used just to maintain this polarization.* This information sends a strong message concerning our eating habits and the choices we make when purchasing our groceries. Quality nutrients provide optimum nutrition in our cells.

FOUR ℘ MIND-BODY HISTORY

The underlying theory and philosophy of mind/body awareness is not new. Many early cultures had their own traditions and laws to maintain the health and prevent the spread of disease.

In the absence of modern scientific methods of measurement, it is noteworthy to observe that ancient cultures supported a general consensus and underlying theme for health and well-being. While it may have appeared primitive to 20th Century medicine, current researchers have uncovered a more scientific basis for the study and validation of earlier health practices such as acupuncture and herbal medicine.

Some early civilizations had an obsession for cleanliness, as demonstrated by the bathing customs of the Egyptians, Greeks, and Romans. Evidence for body balance and healing is found in the writings of Fu Xi around 2953 B.C., who wrote the book on the principles of Chinese medicine and acupuncture. The Chinese believed that the cause of disease was imbalance.

Indian Ayurvedic medical texts date back to around 2500 B.C. It is one of the world's oldest and most complete systems of natural healing, containing great wisdom for all humanity.[178] The system is still in practice today and is often integrated with traditional Western medicine.

Famous physician and teacher of medicine, Hippocrates (468-377 B.C.) founded several medical schools. His theories included balancing the four humors — blood, phlegm, yellow bile, and black bile — through exercise, fresh air, herbs and foods in order to maintain health and ward off sickness.

A new modern day format has emerged in the medical field called *integrative medicine.* Many colleges and universities now offer this education to medical professionals. One program in particular developed by Andrew Weil, MD is at the Arizona Center for Integrative Medicine.[179] There is a National Center for Complementary and Alternative Medicine at The National Institutes of Health in Bethesda, Maryland.

FIVE ࿐ INFLUENCE OF INTENTION

Research at HeartMath have demonstrated that in order to change our health we must also have a clear intention of moving into an emotional state of love and goodwill characterized by what is called *heart coherence*. Heart coherence is a state in which the variability of the heartbeat remains regular. It is necessary for the efficiency of the circulatory and nervous systems. Positive emotions through our thoughts work in harmony with altering our health and happiness.[180]

There is now an abundant of measureable scientific evidence on the positive effects of prayer, meditation, Yoga, exercise, dance and music, and the benefits of whole foods nutrition and its relationship in the recovery of sickness, injuries including cancer. There are instances of unexplainable healing that go beyond the traditional mind of science. The power of collective intention gives rise to a positive mind/body/spirit transformation in the most mysterious of circumstances.

Mind/Body in Cancer

An early pioneer of mind/body medicine is health educator, surgeon, and patient advocate, Bernie Siegel, M.D. During the 1970s at Yale Medical Center he began to organize support groups with his cancer patients. In his first book, *Love, Medicine and Miracles*, he discusses how mind-body medicine was rarely talked about in medical circles. [181] Siegel received peer criticism when he found that by playing music and talking to patients under anesthesia impacted the success of the surgery and rate of recovery. It became readily accepted by his peers with the manifestation of positive results including increase rate of recover.

He studied how dreams were used to interpret a physical illness. Encouraging patients to draw their feelings in the form of art helped him understand their illness and provide a more accurate course of cure. Throughout his research he developed great insight about how events and attitudes create a person's human environment and how they can change their choices.

Siegel's patient support groups practiced transcendental meditation[182], Yoga, prayer, and creative imagery to help control body functions, heart rate, and even reduce/cure cancer. While his peers thought him to be crazy at the time, he also knew that as a physician it was important that he study beyond the scope of what was learned in medical school.

Quantum Leap

Given the enormity of the solar system and the universal realms beyond our planet, the human mind is but a frontier that contains the molecules of possibility only limited by our own small thoughts and experiences. What is truly remarkable is the fact that when we move beyond the ego and limiting thoughts, the mind becomes a prevailing instrument that can be used to alter the future of our self and all human beings. Our beliefs do not just exist in our mind. They become part of a greater consciousness and the infinite probability that direct every molecule, the circadian rhythms[183] of our body, and the universe which ultimately affects the quality of our personal health, the well being of the planet and our future.

SIX ☙ MIND - BODY FUNCTIONAL MEDICINE

When participating in my program, patients are scheduled for return visits. This valuable time is spent in counseling, encouragement and reinforcement. It also includes a few minutes of stepping onto the scale prior to their appointment. It is common to hear sighs of discontent and impatience as the number doesn't always coincide with what a patient thinks it should read. Sometimes there is a quick reverberation of disappointment, occasionally followed with excuses. I've had patients become angry and blame my system.

My response to them is based on my years of experience and the ability to understand their frustration. It also relies on my medical understanding of the human body from years of being a physician. As you can see from reading how powerful the mind/body connection is, the scales are but a small part of the overall program for success.

Patients come from all walks of life, arriving with all of their personal history. Each must be accepted at his or her own level and should be encouraged to practice patience as the body adjusts to a new Lifestyle. Many people have spent years of yo-yo dieting and may have developed habits that just don't serve them as they age. They are often confused from hearing all the so-called theories that are encountered from the day-to-day rhetoric of media or latest gimmick or program for quick weight loss. Even more so, they are fed up with why their past efforts have not worked. The morbid obese have ended up with health issues that have sent them to their doctors. Diagnostic testing and drug therapy become the norm. Dieting in America has created more obesity.

I remind them about why they want to lose weight, their reasons, intentions and desires. One's success, however, relies on his or her commitment to a body/mind tune-up to support his/her continuing success in maintaining a healthy weight and future.

Ultimately, what this is all about is freedom. Learn to step out of your box. Learn to take chances in life, take a risk so that you can grow and be happy.

Support and Laughter

Participating in a positive support system/network helps us through the tough times as well as the celebrations. This support can come from family and friends, our spouse, and spiritual center.

And one very important thought. Laughter releases endorphins that give you a "high". It dissolves disease and it boosts your moral and your immune system. Watch funny movies, tell funny jokes. Laughter is the best medicine. There are no side effects and it is a mini cardio workout.

Laugh loudly, laugh often, and laugh 100 times a day.

ꟸ

V

PATHWAYS TO HEALING AND LONGEVITY

"Aging is essentially a process in which your cells lose their resilience, they lose their ability to repair damage; however, it is within your power to boost that resilience. Our bodies were not designed to fail; they were designed with great efficacy, organization and possess the ability to repair."

E.A. Ordonez, M.D.

ONE ꕤ WELCOME TO AN AGELESS SOCIETY

"Old age will only be respected when it fights for itself, maintains its rights, avoids dependence on anyone, and asserts control over its own to the last breath."

Marcus Tullius Cicero
Roman philosopher, statesman, lawyer
106BC-43BC

Taking care of your health including establishing a healthier weight is your first step toward joining an *ageless society*, a place where ravages of old age, disease, dementia and disability are almost unknown. This ageless society is a place where every man and woman may look forward to a youthful, productive life span of 100 or more years filled with boundless health and unlimited possibility. Advanced progress is being made in almost every area of health. Most far-reaching of all is the fact that we are beginning to conquer mankind's worst nemesis - AGING and DEATH.

How Old Is Old?

Biological factors, not necessarily chronologic ones, determine actual age. Aging is essentially a process by which your cells lose their resilience; they lose their ability to repair damage. As discussed in Part III, we are constantly experiencing free radical activity and oxidative stress that also contributes to aging of the cell's energy source, the mitochondria and the DNA.

Prime physical condition lasts about ten years – age 17-27. A process called sacropenis (*loss of flesh*) begins to decrease muscle tissue and strength by our 30's. At 75, muscle mass reduces to almost half of what it was when we were younger. [184] This occurs as a result of a decrease in the levels of growth hormones, testosterone and other important hormones, which stimulate muscle growth.[185] It is a known fact, however, that individuals can maintain good muscle strength and cognitive (brain) function well into later years through regular exercise.[186]

Biological changes occur with the mitigation of estrogen and other steroid-identified hormones in women. [187] The face and other environmentally exposed areas visibly convey this. Lifestyle, health, sun exposure, activity level, and our thoughts or stress levels all play a vital role at the rate of this process.

Age As A Viewpoint

In Western culture, historical factors, such as moving from the farm to factory to corporate tower, caused great changes in viewpoints and sometimes stigma as more emphasis is place on youth versus old age. The Baby Boomer generation, however, is fighting back. Not too long ago, mandatory age for pilots to retire was 60. It is now 65.[188] Many companies are rehiring retirees to work as consultants. Farmers, academics, doctors, researchers and others could very well work into later years. In other areas of the world such as Costa Rica, a 90-year-old is still working in the fields.[189]

We are also inundated with media advertising for cosmetics and drugs that send negative mixed messages telling us we are going to fall apart tomorrow.

Not too long ago, the traditional medical view has been that AGING is a disease process with inevitable complications and consequences. History has shown that life after 50 and child-bearing years will change dramatically as disease-states take a greater hold of our lives. Our hormones and reduced ability to absorb nutrients will significantly drop off, and life as we knew it, and one in which we took so much for granted, will slowly slip away.

Everything having to do with the ramification of aging and poor lifestyle — heart disease, cancer, diabetes, dementia, obesity, arthritis, including a general steady decline of physical stature, is most disturbing because it results in a decline of the QUALITY of life, including our sex life. It all becomes a faint memory.

TWO ꙮ DON'T GET SICK, DON'T GET OLD, DON'T DIE

Past adages of aging are quickly being replaced with newer paradigms that bring with them a greater understanding of health and longevity. As health care costs become more prohibitive, there is a convergence of integrative methodologies rising up amongst health care professionals. They will eventually override the present conditions of our system. The Baby Boomer generation and their children can no longer stand by and lose their savings and sanity over a dysfunctional structure of health care. This new paradigm shift is PREVENTION. As Benjamin Franklin said, "An ounce of prevention is worth an ounce of cure."

It is the responsibility of every individual to stop relying on someone else to pick up the bill for their carelessness and poor eating and lifestyle habits, including smoking and use of smokeless tobacco, excessive alcohol intake and poor food choices. It is time to deal with the institutions that continue to spend millions of dollars in media advertising telling us that were are going to be sick and that the only way to prevent it is to continue to consume drugs that place a band aid on the real cause behind the disease.

Cost of Health Care

Today in the United States, the Federal Government spends approximately $2.5 trillion dollars, or 17.6% of Gross Domestic Product (GDP) on healthcare.[190] In 1970, these figures were 75 billion for the elderly population with 95% spent on interventional medicine. Actuaries project that by 2010 per capita spending on healthcare for Americans 65+ will $10,000.[191] An *Annals of Internal Medicine* report indicates that heart disease, diabetes, and other chronic diseases underlie the growing burden of adult disability.[192] This accounts for 70% of all deaths in the United States and more than 75% of its $2 trillion cost of medical care.[193]

Within 40 years, Washington will be spending 50% more in healthcare than in Social Security. It is predicted that by 2017-18 the funds for Social Security will be exhausted. By 2075, experts are estimating healthcare expenditures for the elderly to double and stand at 14.5% of GDP.[194]

The Economics of Prevention

When emphasis is placed on PREVENTION we can predict a trend shift and reduction on health care costs. It goes without saying, however, no matter how idealistic, *prevention* is difficult to implement. Purchasing more expensive diagnostic equipment may not be the answer to prevention. Human nature often prevails and it takes a concerted effort to have the general public comply with taking care of their health through simple steps. Compounding this are the socio-economic realities of one's environment.

The focus on prevention requires a paradigm shift that builds the *value* and *benefit* of community-based programs, placing financial resources into the best and simplest methods of prevention. There has to a cooperative effort by health care providers, their patients, and the general public.[195] This requires education. It is estimated that by increasing community health care programs that include exercise, weight loss, improved nutrition, smoking cessation, can reap a savings of $16 billion annually in health care costs.[196] Prevention begins at the earliest age, including infancy, and continues into older age. To save public programs for the senior population requires a public swing that adopts anti-aging medicine as a standard element in the preventive healthcare setting.

Cuts in healthcare spending leave more funds to be appropriated to other public programs. It is the topic of the news and high-ranking officials.

US NEWS & WORLD REPORT

"While politicians are debating how to ration healthcare, scientists are focused on a more promising endeavor alleviating the diseases that commonly come with old age....While there will be many more elderly people, there will not be an increase in chronically disabled elderly.

*Dying old is generally cheaper than dying young. A **70** year old consumes almost three times as much healthcare in the last two years of life as a **101**-year old receives. <u>What is expensive is older people living through years of chronic dependence</u>. Government-funded programs will reap these savings and reduce their tab."*[197]

*"Our current healthcare system is a 'sick care' system with perverse incentives. The disease and economic burden that we have upon us – we currently spend more than $2 trillion per year on health care, or **16%** of our gross domestic product – is largely <u>preventable</u>."*

Richard Carmona, M.D.
Chairperson of Partnership
to Fight Chronic Disease,
former Surgeon General 2002-2006

Financial Benefits of Longevity

An increase of six years in the average life expectancy of total U.S. population achieved **1970-1990** translated into a worth of $57 trillion in **1992** dollars. In the U.S. longevity is worth $2.4 trillion a year.[198]

THREE ℘ ANTI-AGING MEDICINE

Anti-Aging Medicine is a medical specialty founded on the application of advanced scientific and medical technologies for the early detection, prevention, treatment and reversal of age-related dysfunction, disorders, and diseases.

It is a healthcare model promoting innovative science and research to prolong the healthy human lifespan. Anti-aging medicine is based on principles of sound and responsible medical care that are consistent with those applied in other preventive health specialties.

Anti-aging medicine is the application of any therapy or modality that delivers very early detection, prevention, treatment, or reversal of aging-related dysfunction and disease, thus enhancing the quality of life overall.

It is scientific. Evidence-based, anti-aging medicine is supported through an orderly process for acquiring data in order to formulate a scientific and objective assessment upon which an effective treatment is assigned. Anti-aging diagnostic and treatment practices are supported by scientific evidence and therefore cannot be branded as anecdotal.

Anti-aging medicine is supported through the American Academy of Anti-Aging Medicine (A4M) and is consistent with the principles of conventional medicine. It is also well documented by peer-reviewed journals including publications such as *Aging, American Journal of Cardiology,*

Journal of the American Geriatrics Society, and *Journal of the American Medical Association.*

Regenerative Medicine

Anti-aging Medicine IS NOT solely equivalent to Hormone Replacement Therapy or Human Growth Factor HGH). Less than 10% of anti-aging patients receive injectible HGH.

Many anti-aging physicians do indeed prescribe bio-identical hormone replacement and hormonal therapy. They recommend the consumption of quality food and scientifically studied supplements.

Those physicians who have taken a giant leap into the field of integrative medicine support lifestyle changes. This includes weight loss along with improved eating habits to support body regeneration conducive to the age, health and lifestyle of an individual.

The goal of anti-aging medicine is not merely to prolong the total years of an individual's life, but to ensure that those years are enjoyed in a productive and vital fashion. In other words, living longer includes having a quality of life that supports the entire person in the absence of debilitating disease. It is a life in which there is laughter, activity, peace and tranquility filled with music and positive reasons and motivation to greet the morning with joy and enthusiasm. It is a life where one can laugh, sing, and dance well into the night. Dancing sets the chemistry of the mind into motion causing the human machine to function normally.

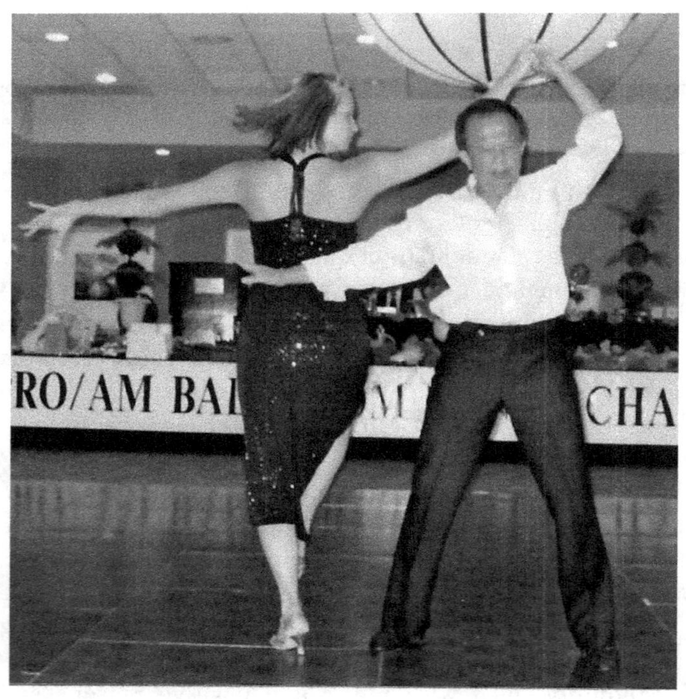
RO/AM BA
CHA

FOUR ☙ PILLARS OF AGING

When assessing the aging process one must realize that there are two significant categories to contemplate. The first is the *chronological* which has to do with our birth date and actual age in years.

The second is our *biological* age, which is a more accurate method of measuring age since it directly reflects what is actually occurring at a cellular level in the biological environment of an individual. It is an accumulative rendering of how we have actually treated our body over the years. Biological aging directly mirrors our thoughts and lifestyle. It echoes our lifetime choices that include the way we think, the food we eat, the air we breathe, the water we drink, our sleep, our health, our daily activities including exercise, and any long term environmental exposure including the sun.

While we cannot turn back the clock we can certainly influence and increase our years and quality of life by reducing risk factors that accelerate biological aging.

Biological markers that increase with age	Biological markers that reduce with age
• Insulin Resistance • Systolic Blood Pressure • Percentage of Body Fat • Lipid Ratios	• Glucose Tolerance • Aerobic Capacity • Muscle Mass • Strength • Temperature Regulation • Immune Function

Hormone Replacement

Replacing the several hormones that diminish with age is the best approach to anti-aging. According to Thiery Hertoghe, MD, a Belgian endocrinologist and Secretary General of the Belgium Medical Association and one of the world's leaders in HRT, "the anti-aging hormones work synergistically."

A Word of Caution: Hormone replacement requires the knowledge of an experienced licensed physician. It must be monitored so that recommended prescribed levels are safe and effective.

FIVE ꘙ HABITS FOR LONGEVITY

Lifestyle habits are paramount for improving the aging process. The body requires adequate rest, nutrition and exercise. Eliminating addictive behaviors such as smoking and excessive alcohol will add years to your life.

Nutrition for Life

The most powerful tool you have to accomplish reduction of each pillar of aging is your diet. Although the concept of calorie restriction is at the cutting edge of anti-aging research, in reality it is essentially how your GRANDMOTHER told you to eat. Her advice consisted of four sound anti-aging principles.

- Eat small meals throughout the day.
- Have some protein at every meal
- Always eat your fruits and vegetables.
- Take your cod-liver oil.

Consumption of foods high in antioxidants reduces cellular disease and the damage from free radicals (oxidative stress). Free radicals are highly reactive bits of molecules formed during the process of converting oxygen and food into energy. Like tiny exploding grenades, they can damage cells and the DNA. Thousands of studies support the idea that free radical damage and contributes to age-related illnesses.

Exercise — A Hormone-Altering "Drug"

Exercise is a powerful anti-aging prescription. People who are physically fit, eat a healthy balanced diet, and take nutritional supplements can slice 10 to 20 years off their biological age. True body age should be measured in terms of FUNCTION.

Does exercise make you live longer? Yes and no. If you are purely sedentary, any type of exercise will increase your life span up to a point. It doesn't matter what type of exercise you do as long as you burn about 300 calories per day. The benefits are astounding!

Medical Dancing for Health – The Functional Medicine

Dancing is a powerful form of exercise and has numerous benefits.

- Dancing releases neurotransmitter hormones that make you HIGH as you dance the night away.
- Energizes and motivates with the rhythm music.
- Takes away the present circumstances and lifts us into the beauty of possibility and creativity.
- Helps us to heal and feel more balanced.
- Births hope for change and enhancements in our relationships.

- Music and rhythm lives on when everything else appears to be dying around us. It gives us wings to fly higher when tragedy pulls us into the path of despair.
- Is fun, adds meaning and quality to life.
- It is a current in the ocean of life moving us towards the Place of our Dreams.
- Dance contributes to increased confidence and self-esteem.
- Dance contributes to good posture and body alignment preventing osteoporosis.
- Increases flexibility, stamina and endurance.
- Ultimately all the unwanted body fats vanish with the reduction of excess weight.

Out of sixty forms of physical activities studied, dancing ranks in the top five. So why not dance to the Music of the Heart, the Mind, the Body, and the Soul. You will look younger, feel better, and live longer. Your biological clock beats to your personal experience of time — reversing the aging process. Personally, it is the best leveraging factor that's worth living for.

Words for Reflection

QUESTION: What's more invasive than a computer virus and far more difficult to get rid of?

ANSWER: AGING

Think about it. We do plenty to prevent our computer from crashing. We feed it new software to improve functionality. We give it upgrades, improve its memory, and install virus protection to ensure our data won't suffer any serious damage.

A growing number of scientists are bewildered. They want to know why we aren't paying as much attention to our own "hardware". They now know that prevention plays a vital role. It is required to properly drive the critical systems in our bodies.

The body experiences changes as we grow older. Time alone is not responsible for eroding health. This means the damaging effects of age may not be inevitable. Advances in medical science have provided treatments that delay, prevent and in some cases reverse the diseases and ailments associated with aging. Why not make it our business by staying healthy?

ଔ

VI

MIND-BODY-BEAUTY

"Beauty is more than skin deep. Within the very essence of each cell resides the potential to resonate and bring forth light and health for the future."

Alexandra J. Zani

ঔ৶

ONE ℘ MORE THAN SKIN DEEP

"Fashion is not something that exists in dresses only. Fashion is in the sky, in the street; fashion has to do with ideas, the way we live, what is happening."

Gabrielle Bonheur "Coco" Chanel, Couturière, 1883-1971

The process of losing weight goes beyond the realm of reaching one's goals. It's about taking this time to redesign your life, your future, and how you want to live and be in the world. When you are healthy there is a feeling of elation and beauty. You are filled with confidence that indeed you are able to achieve something greater than what was thought possible.

It is also a good time to do some special things just for you to help ease the weight loss process and prevent stress. Take 10 minutes of quiet time or a brief walk in nature twice daily; have a relaxing massage or facial at your favorite spa. You can also invest in a series of body sculpting treatments to expedite your weight loss process.

Physiological Alterations

While there are wonderful internal enhancements occurring during a course of weight reduction, you may notice that your skin begins to sag. If you have carried around extra pounds for years, the muscles may have weakened and the underlying skin structures are probably not as healthy. Lack of proper exercise and/or yo-yo dieting through eating too few calories causes the body to lose muscle mass and damage the cells' ability to repair.

Additionally, excessive sun exposure or tanning beds will cause premature skin aging since it damages DNA and other cell structures. Lifestyle habits including smoking will cause premature aging.[199]

The skin is an elastic tissue that requires optimum nutrition to build good collagen in the underlying skin structures. It has the ability to extend, as certainly experienced during pregnancy. Losing weight too fast may be counterproductive in having your skin shrink to your new body.

Extra weight causes the skin to stretch. It doesn't always "spring back" after losing the pounds. Moreover, new mothers may experience stretch marks from childbirth or excess sagging skin.

A gradual weight loss allows the skin to adjust to your new size. Reaching your ideal weight requires that you consume enough healthy calories each day in order to reconstruct new muscle and tissue. Muscle mass can be rebuilt through good nutrition and weight bearing exercise while decreasing fat. This process is very individual and varies with each person. It may be beneficial to consult with an exercise physiologist or personal trainer who can direct a customized exercise routine for you.[200]

TWO ꟾ NEW TECHNOLOGY

We are fortunate to have the latest technology available to assist in enhancing our appearance during and after the weight loss process. Along with good nutrition, there are skin treatments and home care regimens to support the integrity of the skin.

A newer generation of skin care products called *cosmeceuticals*, contain performance ingredients that actually do something to enhance the skin's appearance. In-clinic facial and body treatments help support circulation and diminish stress and the signs of aging.[201,202]

Light Technologies for Skin Rejuvenation

Lasers/IPL

Lasers have been used for years in medicine for assisting physicians in surgery and in ophthalmology. A newer generation of lasers called *aesthetic lasers* proves to be less invasive and have the ability to reduce hair, stimulate the skin's collagen production resulting in firmer skin, and reduce the appearance of pigmentation and spider veins.[203,204] Some of the latest lasers are designed to specifically address spot fat reduction and body contouring.[205]

LED (Light-Emitting Diode or Bio-photo-modulation) Therapy

Initially developed for wound healing for astronauts living in a non-gravitational environment, LED therapy is now used for improvement of skin conditions. A non-invasive treatment called bio-photo-modulation therapy uses pure wave-lengths of light to rejuvenate the skin. In aesthetic medicine, specific wavelengths of color are applied to treat wrinkles, pigment, support circulation, reduce inflammation and even treat acne.

LED therapy was developed for astronauts during space flight. Wounds heal slowly in a microgravity environment. Additionally, the Medical College of Wisconsin as well as other universities are studying how LED therapy can support healing of wounds from diabetic skin ulcers and serious burns.[206,207]

What is the difference between a laser and an LED? Lasers and other devices (radio frequency as in Thermage® and others) use heat through a process called *controlled wounding* (collagen contraction for skin tightening) or *selective photothermolysis* (for hair reduction). This process can destroy a hair follicle (as in hair reduction) or cause tissue (collagen) contraction, resulting in skin tightening.

LED or bio-photo-modulation therapy stimulates biological tissue non-invasively without heating. It stimulates tissue repair, tissue tightening, and can also treat pigment and acne. The devices are FDA registered and are less expensive than a laser or IPL device. It is a great therapy to be used in conjunction with the new micro current machines. Note that LEDs are not used for hair reduction.

Microcurrent Technology

Not ready for the laser? Recent innovative treatments include the use of microcurrents, which have been used worldwide in wound healing, in sports medicine and tissue rebuilding from injury[208],[209]. They are also used in equestrian and veterinary centers in Great Britain, the United States and Canada.

Microcurrent technology is now available in the aesthetic industry. It is used to perform non invasive lifts for face, breast, abdominals, and upper legs and is effective in scar repair/reduction.

Microcurrents are the natural energy that is found in your body and are responsible for muscle movement and other chemical electric impulse processes. When applied in sports injuries they help augment the body's own healing ability. Microcurrents are also used in pain and disease management.

Numerous studies have been shown that application of microcurrent can help tissue to heal 500% faster than by conventional methods. In aesthetic medicine they help with skin and muscle rejuvenation and are used pre/post surgically to help with healing and reduce inflammation. [210,211]

Injectibles and fillers

Botox Cosmetic®[212] and other dermal fillers have flooded the marketplace in the rush to defy wrinkles. It is recommended that a reputable physician perform the procedures.

The Future

The future is definitely linked to the bridging of both traditional medicine and prevention modalities that are joined together to offer aesthetic enhancements focused on the health and wellbeing of an individual. The spa and wellness fields have existed together for a long time and will continue to do so as we direct our efforts towards prevention.

During the mid-1990s, there was a tremendous surge of interest from many medical practitioners to bring more innovative modalities into their practices. Complimentary and ancillary services support patients who seek professional intervention when it comes to slowing the aging process including cancer prevention.

The body cannot be segmented. Its beauty and vitality lie deep within each cell and the Mind that governs it. The skin and what is underneath will always be a showcase of our very existence and lifestyle.

NOTHING TASTES AS GOOD AS THIN FEELS!

A Sampling

of

Our Success Stories

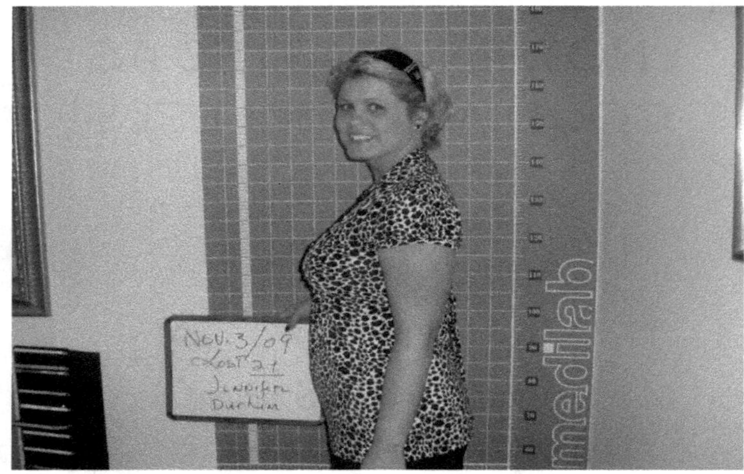

I have been seeing Dr. O for about 4 months, I have lost about 30 pounds and feel incredible. I never thought I would be able to fit into my 16-yr-old's clothes. We are now fighting about who gets to wear what each day. What a great problem to have.

I have been getting tons of compliments from family, friends and co-workers. But the one that takes the cake is when I took my 11th grade daughter to her school orientation. I met her teachers and even some of her friends. The next day, my daughter tells me that her teachers thought I was her older sister, not her mom. Then she tells me that one of her guy friends said, "Your Mom is hot!" I have not had that kind of compliment in a long time.

Thanks, Dr. O, I couldn't do this without you!!! ***Jennifer Durham, 1/06/2010***

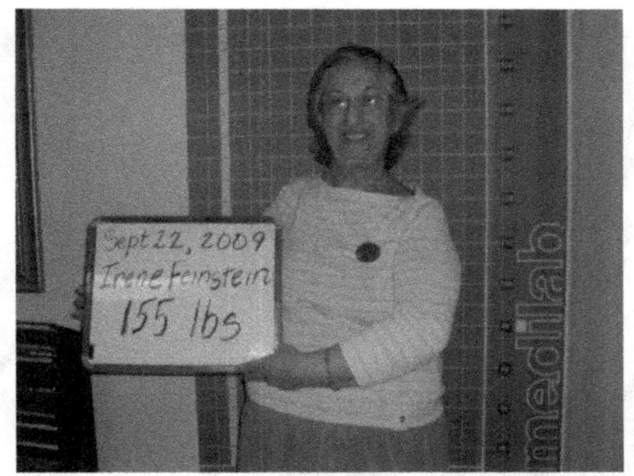

Irene Feinstein, went from an initial 196 lbs down to 146 lbs by Dec 17, 2009

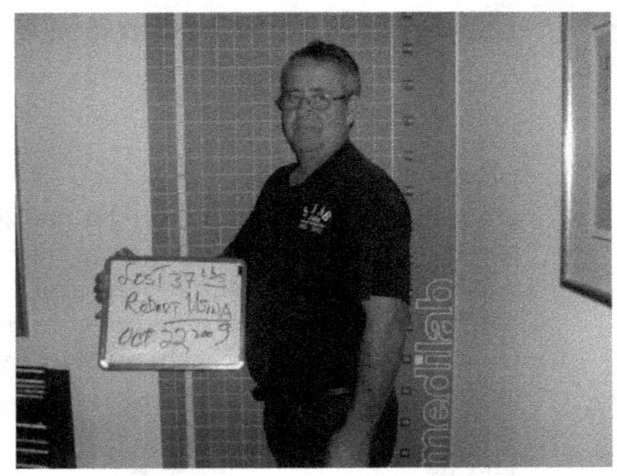

Robert Usina lost 37 lbs

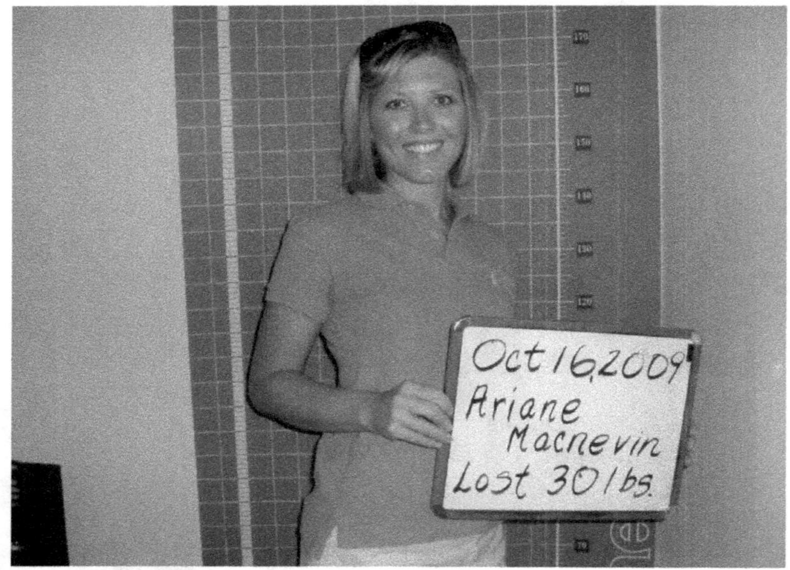

Doctor Ordoñez has changed my life in so many ways. I feel great and look amazing. He has taught me to make healthy lifestyle choices that have made me a better wife and mother. I am more active now and owe it to him and his staff for their wonderful support in my journey to get fit but most of all healthy. **Nothing will ever taste as good as skinny feels**.

Thank you,

Ariane MacNevin

"I started my journey to a healthier me when I reached a weight of 225 lbs and I wanted to look and feel better.....I sat down with Dr. O and he asked me how he could help me reach my goals. I told him I wanted to be able to run again....I left with a meal plan, two prescriptions, a better understanding of self and a new motivation that I had not had before. My process has been slow and steady over the year and as of my last visit I weighed 169.5 lbs. But I gained a mentor, a motivator and have been blessed to meet one of the most genuine gentlemen I have ever known."

—S.D. Mercer

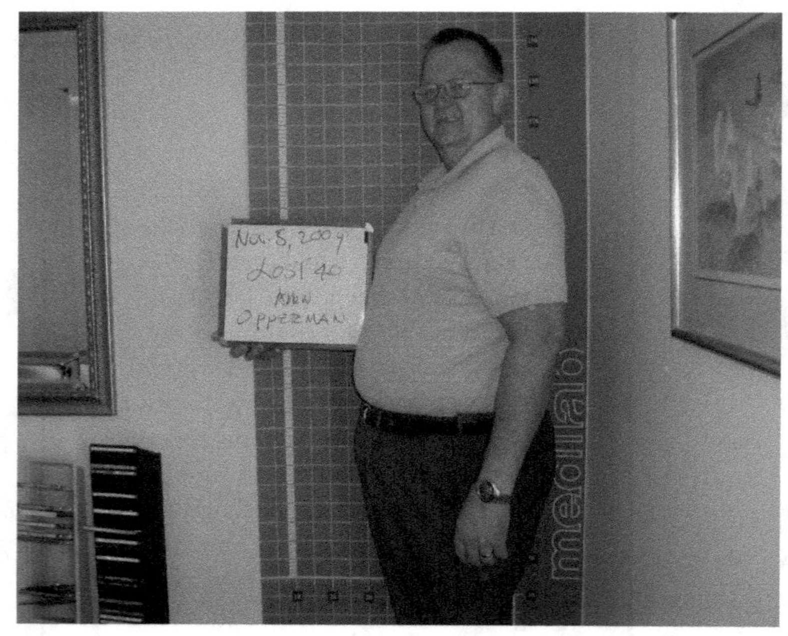

Allen Opperman lost 40 lbs total

YOU CAN, TOO!!

About the Authors

Ernesto A. Ordoñez, MD

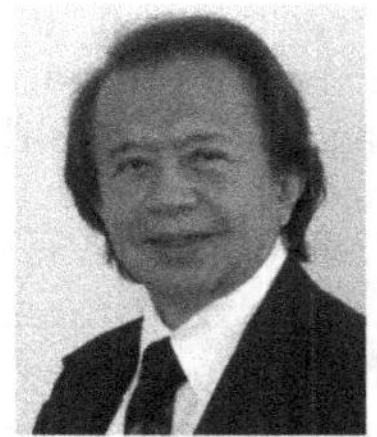

Dr. Ordoñez is a graduate of the University of Santo Tomas College of Medicine and Surgery, Manila, Philippines and did his internship/residency training in Ohio. His memberships and affiliations include

- Philippine Medical Society of Northeast Florida
- Member of the American Academy of Anti-Aging Medicine since 1997
- Served as Chairman of Family practice for local hospitals
- Past Major in the U.S. Air Force Reserve —conducted Wellness Programs

Dr. Ordoñez owns and operates The Centre for Weight Loss, Regenerative and Aesthetic Medicine in Jacksonville, Florida His center encompasses an innovative concept for the achievement of optimum weight loss, health and well being. He has a passion to help people achieve a healthy lifestyle in order to prevent the damaging effects of obesity/overweight and the burden of "old age". Optimal wellness — a mind, body, spirit approach:

1. Weight Management and Lifestyle Change
2. Medical Age Management (Nutrition, Bio-identical hormones, HGH).
3. Advanced Aesthetics for face and body (including body sculpting through advanced technology)
4. Stress Reduction

5. Medical Dancing – for a healthier mind and body and improving the quality of life.
6. Education & Research – Education brings value and understanding for Lifestyle Transformation.

Breaking through the barriers of traditional weight loss treatment ideas, the center closely interacts with its guests to plan a scientifically sound program to support their unique requirements for maintaining optimal wellness. Dr. Ordoñez personally interviews each individual where they team together to develop personal goals and commitment levels. Personal success continues throughout scheduled visits and monthly educational seminars. A key to Dr. Ordoñez' success is the one-on-one motivational session scheduled throughout the weight loss program. Lifetime management is an ultimate objective for each guest. After they reach their goal, they are welcome to schedule future visits to re-affirm their health objectives and commitment.

The heartbeat of success in this program is positive support — COUNSELING, ENCOURAGEMENT and REINFORCE- MENT. Additionally, adjunctive therapy such as the use of appetite suppressants helps with this transformational process.

Alexandra J. Zani

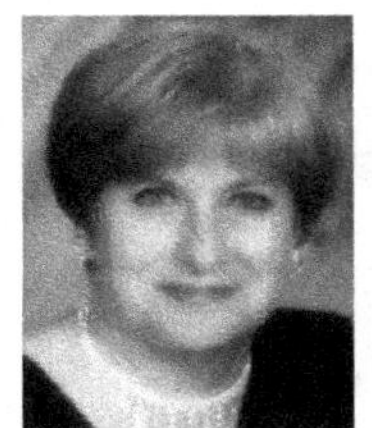

An international educator, Alexandra Zani is a licensed cosmetologist /esthetician, independent technical consultant and scientific advisor for post-graduate studies in the medical spa industry. Her education background includes biology and medical technology. Zani is a specialist in the anti-aging sciences, including the affects of nutrition, lifestyle and the mind/body connection. She writes curriculum for non-ablative lasers, microcurrent, LED, microdermabrasion, and related aesthetic modalities for anti-aging.

Ms. Zani has studied and received numerous certifications in her field of expertise. She is currently nationally certified through NCEA, (National Coalition of Estheticians, Manufacturers/Distributors Associations) and was recognized as a five-star educator through the American Aestheticians Education Association (former AAEA). Zani has published in Cosmetic Dermatology Times, beauty New Zealand, Les Nouvelles Esthetique (U.S edition), and Dermascope Magazine. She was lead author for 2003 *Milady's Standard Comprehensive Training for Estheticians*, and a contributing author in *Advanced Professional Skin Care – Medical Edition*, by Peter T. Pugliese, M.D. A cosmeceutical formulation specialist, she develops line synergies and produces technical writing and support.

REFERENCE NOTES

Notes — Introduction

[1] Center for Chronic Disease Prevention and Health Promotion, Overweight and Obesity, Retrieved from www.ced.gov/obesity/data/index.html

[2]Flegal KM, Carroll MD, Ogden CL, Curtin LR. Prevalence and trends in obesity among US adults, 1999-2008. *JAMA* 2010: DOI: 10.1001/jama.2009.2014. Retrieved from http://www.jama.com.

[3] O'Riordan, M (2010, January 13) Most American Overweight, and One-Third Are Obese: HANES. Retrieved from Heartwire, www.medscape.com/viewarticle/715051_print

[4] Doane, Seth, (2010, January 7). CBS News: *Where America Stands* series. Battling Obesity in America. Retrieved from http://www.cbsnews.com/stories/2010/01/07/eveningnews/main6069163.shtml

Notes —C II:

---

[5] Ionamin is a registered trademark of Celltech Pharmaceuticals, Inc. Pondimin is a registered trademark of Robins Pharmaceuticals.

[6] Benjamin, R.M. MD. The Surgeon General's Vision for a Healthy and Fit Nation (February 2010), Retrieved from http://www.surgeongeneral.gov/library/obesityvision/obesityvision2010.pdf

[7] Spurlock, M. (2004) *Super-Size Me.* CD Available from Amazon.com

[8] Streib, L. (2008, February 8) World's Fattest Countries. Forbes Magazine. Retrieved from http://www.forbes.com/2007/02/07/worlds-fattest-countries-forbeslife-cx_ls_0208worldfat_print.html

---

[9] Thomson, T.G. (2002, June 20) Human Health Services. Retrieved from htt;://seniorjournal.com/NEWS/Fitness/2-06-20-300MDie.htm

[10] Center for Disease Control (2010) Division of Nutrition, Physical Activity and Obesity, National Center for Chronic Disease Prevention and Health Promotion. Retrieved from http://www.cdc.gov/obesity/data/index.html

[11]Karlgard, R. (2009, July 9) Digital Rules, Our Health Care Crisis: Age, Obesity, Lawyers Retrieved from http://www.forbes.com/forbes/2009/0907/opinions-rich-karlgaard-digital-rules_print.html

[12] Statistics Related to Overweight and Obesity (2007, June) National Institute of Diabetes and Digestive and Kidney Diseases. Retrieved from http://win.niddk.nih.gov/publications/PDFs/stat904z.pdf

[13] Taeku, L and Olive, J.E. Public Opinions and Weight Action About Diet, Nutrition and Physical Activity. Americans Attitudes About Overweight. Retrieved from http://www.libraryindex.com/pages/2765/Public-Opinion-Action-About-Diet-Weight-Nutrition-Physical-Activity-AMERICANS-ATTITUDES-ABOUT-OVERWEIGHT.html

[14] Kirshenbaum, D. PhD (2008) Obesity Treatment. Misguided Diplomacy: Getting Past the "Fear" of Telling a Child They Are Overweight or Obese Retrieved from http://www.obesity-treatment.com/content/misguided-diplomacy-getting-past-fear-telling-a-child-they-are-overweight-or-obese?referrer

[15] American Academy of Pediatrics. Prevention of Pediatric Overweight and Obesity: American Academy of Pediatrics Policy Statement; Organizational Principles to Guide and Define the Child Health System and/or Improve the Health of All Children; Committee on Nutrition. *Pediatrics.* 2003;112:424-430

[16] Whitaker RC, Wright JA, Pepe MS, Seidel KD, Dietz WH. Predicting obesity in young adulthood from childhood and parental obesity. *N Engl J Med* 1997; 37(13):869–873.

[17] Kistler, K.D., et al. (2010, February) Alimentary Pharmacology & Therapeutics. 2010;31(3):396-406. Retrieved from (http://www.medscape.com/viewarticle/715147?src=mp&spon=20&uac=27838SZ

[18] Facts for Families (2008, May) Obesity in Children and Teens. American Academy of Child and Adolescent Psychiatry, 79.
[19] IBID

[20] Brennan, D and Carpenter, C (2009, March) Proximity of Fast-Food Restaurants to Schools and Adolescent Obesity. *American Journal of Public Health*, 99:3.

[21] Healthy Youth. Childhood Obesity (2010) National Center for Disease Prevention and Health Promotion. Retrieved from http://www.cdc.gov/HealthyYouth/obesity/

Notes — C III:

[22] NHANES data on the Prevalence of Overweight Among Children and Adolescents: United States, 2003–2006. CDC National Center for Health Statistics, Health E-Stat.

[23] Barclay, Laurie MD (2010, January 28) Overweight Elderly Have similar Mortality to Normal-Weight Elderly. Retrieved from http://www.medscape.com/viewarticle/716067?src=mp&spon=20&uac=27838SZ

[24] U.S. Census Bureau, Population Profile of the United States. Retrieved from http://www.census.gov/population/www/pop-profile/natproj.html

[25] Brikey, M. PhD (2000) *Defy Aging: Develop the Mental and Emotional Vitality to Live Longer, Healthier, and Happier Than You Ever Imagined* (p. 3) New Resources Press, Columbus, OH.

[26] *Clinical Guidelines on the Identification, Evaluation, and Treatment of Overweight and Obesity in Adults,* NHLBI, September 1998.

[27] Hellmich, Nanci (2009) Rising obesity will cost U.S. health care $344 billion a year. USA Today. Retrieved from http://www.usatoday.com/news/health/weightloss/2009-11-17-future-obesity-costs_N.htm

---

[28] Hicks, J. (2008, November 4) A Sedentary Lifestyle and Diabetes. Retreived from http://diabetes.about.com/od/benefitsofexercise/a/sedentary7.htm?p=1

[29] Booth, FW, Chakravarthy, M. (2002, March) Cost and Consequences of Sedentary Living: New Battleground for an Old Enemy. Research Digest, President's Council on Physical Fitness and Sports. Retrieved from http://www.fitness.gov/researchdigestmarch2002.pdf

[30] Nerenberg, L. (2002) Caregiver Stress and Elder Abuse. National Institute on Aging, National Center on Elder Abuse, San Francisco, California Retrieved from http://www.ncea.aoa.gov/Main_Site/pdf/family/caregiver.pdf

[31] Barclay, Laurie MD (2010, January 28) Overweight Elderly Have similar Mortality to Normal-Weight Elderly. Retrieved from http://www.medscape.com/viewarticle/716067?src=mp&spon=20&uac=27838SZ

[32] Booth, FW, Chakravarthy, M. (2002, March) Cost and Consequences of Sedentary Living: New Battleground for an Old Enemy (2002) Presidents Council on Physical Fitness and Sports. Pg. 2. Retrieved from http://www.fitness.gov/researchdigestmarch2002.pdf

[33] Beyond Health Care: New Directions to a Healthier America (2009) Robert Wood Johnson Foundation, Commission to Build a Healthier America. Pg. 8

[34] A Call to Action for Individuals & their Communities. (2009) Americas Health Rankings. 116 pages. Retrieved from http://www.americashealthrankings.org/2009/report/AHR2009%20Final%20Report.pdf

[35] Barish, G.D., Narkar, V.A., Evans, R.M. (2006, March) ***PPARδ***: a dagger in the heart of the metabolic syndrome. *J. Clin. Invest.* **116**(3): 590-597 (2006). doi:10.1172/JCI27955. Retrieved from http://www.jci.org/articles/view/27955

[36] Longley, R. (2003) Obesity, Diabetes on the Increase in the U.S. Retrieved from http://usgovinfo.about.com/library/weekly/aa010803a.htm?p=1

Notes — C IV:

[37] **Adelle Davis (1904-1974)** was an American pioneer in the fledgling field of nutrition during the mid-20th century. She promoted whole unprocessed foods, criticized food additives, and claimed that dietary supplements and other nutrients play a dominant role maintaining health, preventing disease, and restoring health after the onset of disease:

"Research shows that diseases of almost every variety can be produced by an under-supply of various combinations of nutrients... can be corrected when all nutrients are supplied, provided irreparable damage has not been done; and, still better, that these diseases can be prevented." Davis, Adelle (1985)*Let's Have Healthy Children* Available through Amazon.com

[38] Price, Weston A. *(2008) Nutrition and Physical Degeneration.* Price-Pottenger Foundation, 6th Edition.

[39] Byrnes, S. ND, PhD,RNCP, Vegetarian Myths. Posted April 20, 2000, Mercola.com. Retrieved from http://articles.mercola.com/sites/articles/archive/2000/04/02/vegetarian-myths.aspx

[40] Price, Weston A. *(2008) Nutrition and Physical Degeneration.* Price-Pottenger Foundation, 6th Edition.

[41] Fallon-Morell, Sally (2008, October) Twenty-eighth Annual E.F. Schumacher Lecture. The E. F. Schumacher Society. http://www.smallisbeautiful.org/publications/fallon-morell.html

[42] Jones, Desiree, PhD. (2009, October) Heart Disease, Cancer, and Diabetes – What's (Sustainable) Food Got To Do With It? Retrieved from http://www.wellsphere.com/health-education-article/heart-disease-cancer-and-diabetes-what-s-sustainable-food-got-to-do-with-it/828802

[43] Pollan, M. (2008) *In Defense of Food, An Eater's Manifesto.* 2:96-97.

[44] Vokshoor, A.,MD, McGregor, J. MD (2008) Anatomy of the Olfactory System. *eMedicine* Retrieved from http://emedicine.medscape.com/article/835585-print

---

[45] Weil, A. (2008, March 27) Unami: What's That Great Taste? Retrieved from http://www.drweil.com/drw/u/QAA400377/Umami-Whats-That-Great-Taste.html

[46] Jacobs DR Jr, Meyer KA, Kushi LH, Folsom AR. Is whole grain intake associated with reduced total and cause-specific death rates in older women? The Iowa Women's Health Study. *Am J Public Health* 1999;89:322-9

[47] Prevention and Etiology Research Program Iowa Women's Healthy Study. Masonic Cancer Center of the University of Minnesota. Retrieved from http://www.cancer.umn.edu/research/programs/peiowa.html

[48] Jacobs, D.R., Steffen, L.M. (2003) Nutrients, foods, and dietary patterns as exposures in research: a framework for food synergy. *Am J Clin Nutr* 78(suppl): 508S-13S. Retrieved from www.ajcn.org

[49] Ibid

[50] Ackerman, J. (2002, May) Biotech Foods, Science and Space. National Geographic. Retrieved from http://science.nationalgeographic.com/science/article/food-how-altered.html

[51] Domingo, J.L. (2000) Health risks of genetically modified foods: Many opinions but few data. *Science* 288, 1748-1749.

[52] Ackerman, IBID

[53] Vartan, Starre (2006, Nov/Dec) Ah-tchoo! Do Genetically Modified Foods Cause Allergies? Retrieved from http://www.emagazine.com/view/?3427&printview

[54] Séralini, G. E., Spiroux de Vendômois, J., Cellier, D. et al (2009) How Subchronic and Chronic Health Effects can be Neglected for GMOs, Pesticides or Chemicals. *Int J Biol Sci* 2009; 5:438-443 ©Ivyspring International Publisher. Retrieved from http://www.biolsci.org/v05p0438.htm

[55] Pusztai, Arpad (2001) Genetically Modified Foods. Actionbioscience.org. Retrieved from http://www.actionbioscience.org/biotech/pusztai.html

[56] Pollan, M. (2008) *In Defense of Food, An Eater's Manifesto.* 2:101-102.

[57] Fallon, Sally (1999, 2001). *Nourishing Traditions: The Cookbook that Challenges Politically Correct Nutrition and the Diet Dictocrats.* New Trends Publishing, Inc. Washington, DC.

[58] The Weston Price Foundation Newsletter (2005, Dec. 26) Dirty Secrets of the Food Processing Industry. Retrieved from http://www.westonaprice.org/Dirty-Secrets-of-the-Food-Processing-Industry.html

[59] U.S. Census Bureau (2007, March 27) Single-Parent Households Showed Little Variation Since 1994, Census Bureau Reports. Retrieved from http://www.census.gov/Press-Release/www/releases/archives/families_households/009842.html

[60] Kirsch, I., Jungebult. A. et al. (2002, April) Adult Literacy in American: A First Look at the Findings of the National Adult Literacy Survey. U.S. Dept. of Education Office of Educational Research and Improvement NCES 1993-275. Retrieved from http://nces.ed.gov/pubs93/93275.pdf

[61] Drewnowski, A. (2005, August 15) Researchers Find Link Strong Link Between Obesity, Poverty; Healthy Foods Too Costly for Many, Experts Say. redOrbit Knowledge Network. Retrieved from http://www.redorbit.com/news/health/208843/researchers_find_strong_link_between_obesity_poverty_healthy_foods_too/#

[62] Strasser, J.A., Damresh, S., Gaines, J. (1991) Nutrition and the Homeless Person. J Com Health Nur Vol 8, No. 2. (pp 65-73)

[63] Campaign for Commercial-Free Childhood (2005, July 7) Food Marketing to Kids Workshop – Comment, Project No. P034519. pp 2-5. Retrieved from http://www.ftc.gov/os/comments/FoodMarketingtoKids/516960-00053.pdf

[64] Fulton, A. (March 30, 2011) FDA Probes Link Between Food Dyes, Kids' Behavior. Retrieved from www.npr.org/2011/03/30/134962888/fda-probes-link-between-food-dyes-kids-behavior

[65] Anderson, Mike (2009) Documentary: Eating. 3rd Edition. Available through Amazon.com

[66] http://www.bruceames.org/

[67] Markheim, D., Riedl, B. (2007, Feb 5) Farm Subsidies, Free Tarde, and the Doha Round. Retrieved from http://www.heritage.org/RESEARCH/BUDGET/wm1337.cfm

[68] Johnson, Patrick (2008, December 3) U.S. Farm Policy: Subsidizing Poor Health. Retrieved from http://www.heritage.org/Research/Agriculture/wp032609b.cfm

[69] Grandon, T., Deesing, M. (2008) Humane Livestock Handling. Storey Publishing, No. Adams, MA. Pp 33-34

[70] Schlosser, Eric (2001, January 18) American Are Obsessed with Fast Food: The Dark Side of the All-American Meal. CBS Health Watch. Retrieved from http://www.cbsnews.com/stories/2002/01/31/health/main326858.shtml

[71] Motavalli, J. (January/February 2002) The Case Against Meat: Evidence Shows that Our Meat-Based Diet is Bad for the Environment, Aggravates Global Hunger, Brutalizes Animals and Compromises our Health. Environmental Magazine. Retrieved from http://www.emagazine.com/view/?142

[72] Philipott, T. (2010, Feb 23) New research: synthetic nitrogen destroys soil carbon, underminds health http://www.grist.org/article/2010-02-23-new-research-synthetic-nitrogen-destroys-soil-carbon-undermines-/

[73] South Korea, EU, FTA indicates that European Beef Imports may resume. Retrieved from http://www.bilaterals.org/article.php3?id_article=16120

[74] Beck, Saul (2005, December 1) Study reveals U.S. beef consumption statistics by age, income, gender, race, etc. Frozen Food Digest
Retrieved from http://www.allbusiness.com/manufacturing/food-manufacturing-fruit/852845-1.html

[75] American Beef: Why is it Banned in Europe? Retrieved from http://medicine.org/american-beef-why-is-it-banned-in-europe/

[76] Ocean Link, Bamfield Marine Sciences Centre, British Columbia. Retrieved from http://oceanlink.island.net/biodiversity/ask/algae.html

[77] The Rising Tides of Ocean Plagues (2006, April 1) The Science Show. Retrieved from http://www.abc.net.au/rn/scienceshow/stories/2006/1601604.htm
[78] Forristal, Joyce (2000, June 12)The Great Salmon Scam. In sight on The News. Retrieved from http://findarticles.com/p/articles/mi_m1571/is_22_16/ai_62741745/

[79] Pollen, Michael, (2007, January 28) Unhappy Meals. New York Times, 14 pgs. Retrieved from http://www.nytimes.com/2007/01/28/magazine/28nutritionism.t.html?pagewanted=print

[80] Buettner, D. (n.d.) How Blue Zone Works http://www.bluezones.com/

[81] The World Health Organization Retrieved from http://www.who.int/whr/2000/media_centre/press_release/en/print.html

[82] Health Effects of Obesity Fact Sheet, American Obesity Association Retrieved from http://obesity1.tempdomainname.com/subs/fastfacts/Health_Effects.shtml

[83] Centers for Disease Control

[84] IBID, See citation 47

[85] Oldways Past Events. Retrieved from http://www.oldwayspt.org/eventsandtours/pastevents

[86] Nutrients, foods, and dietary patterns as exposure in research: a framework for food synergy (2010) *Am J Clin Nutr* 2003;78 (suppl): 508S-13S. Retrieved from www.ajcn.org

[87] Lyon Diet Heart Study (n.d.) American Heart Association. Retrieved from http://www.americanheart.org/presenter.jhtml?identifier=4655

[88] Mediterranean Diet: Choose this heart-healthy diet options (n.d.). Retrieved from http://www.mayoclinic.com/health/mediterranean-diet/CL00011

---

[89] Heber, D. MD, Bowerman, S. (2001) What Color Is Your Diet? Harper Collins. (p. 8-10)

[90] What is Cancer? (2009, May 11) National Cancer Institute. Retrieved from http://www.cancer.gov/cancertopics/what-is-cancer/print?page=&keyword=

[91] Lyon Diet Heart Study (n.d.) American Heart Association. Retrieved from http://www.americanheart.org/presenter.jhtml?identifier=4655

[92] Southern states tops for heart disease (2007, February 15), CNBC. Retrieved March 2010 from http://www.msnbc.msn.com/id/17170134/
[93] IBID see 49

[94] The Acid Alkaline Balance: The key to vibrant health (February 1, 2009) Wolfe Clinic Newsletter, Kelowna, Canada. Retrieved from http://www.thewolfeclinic.com/newsletters/2009/february/the_acid_alkaline_balance.html

[95] Pugliese, P.T.,MD (2005) Advanced Professional Skin Care , Medical Edition. The Topical Agent, Bernville, PA. pp. 245-246.

[96]Masquelier, Jack Arthur, PhD. (1922-2009) was involved in both phytochemistry and human health. He produced the original research on oligomeric proanthocyanidins (OPCs) in 1948 in a doctorate thesis upon the successful isolation and chemical description of OPCs. He developed a method of extraction to isolate OPCs from both maritime pine bark extract and grapes. OPCs contain very high in antioxidants and have the ability to neutralize free radicals, which are the common cause of numerous diseases.

Pycnogennol (*Pinus pinaster* ssp. Atlantica): French maritime pine contains oligomeric proanthocyanidins (OPCs) as well as several other bioflavonoids: catechin, epicatechin, phenolic fruit acids (such as ferulic acid and caffeic acid), and taxifolin. Procyanadins are oligomeric catechins found at high concentrations in red wine, grapes, cocoa, cranberries, applies, and some supplements such as Pycnogenol® Research includes studies on ADHD, Diabetes, chronic venous insufficiency, asthma, high blood pressure, high cholesterol, melasma, and reduction of platelet aggregation. www.nlm.nih.gov/medineplus/druginfo/natural/patient-pycnogenol.html

[97] Hartle, D.K., Greenspan, P., Hargrove, J.L. (2008) Muscadine Health: Healthful Benefits of Muscadine Products. Blue Heron Nutraceuticals, St. George Island, FL 32328, pp 4-5.

[98] Sinclair, D. et al (2003) Small Molecule Increases Lifespan and "Healthspan" of Obese Mise". Retrieved from http://web.med.harvard.edu/sites/RELEASES/html/11_1Sinclair.html

[99] Hartle, D. K., Greenspan, P., Hargrove, J.L. (2008) Muscadine Health: Health Benefits of Muscadine Products. Blue Heron Nutraceuticals, LLC.

[100]The ORAC value (Oxygen Radical Absorbance Capacity) of one cup of a Heartland Select™ muscadine blend that contains the skin, pulp and seed, contains about 15,000 ORAC units of antioxidants or approximately 4000 ORAC units per two ounces. Additionally, this powerful juice is a product of American farms and is not imported.

[101] Harder, R. (2001, October) The Power of Enzymes. http://www.defeatcancer.ca, Retrieved from http://thyroid.about.com/library/news/blenzymes.htm

[102] A Graphic depiction of the importance of Amylase in Cancer-immuno-enzyme therapy – John Beard
A page that provides the images that show how the carbohydrates surrounding the cancer cell mask the proteins embedded in the cell from attack by protein digesting enzymes. Most enzyme therapies today focus on these proteinases and neglect amylase. In the suffusing form of this coating, the hormone hCG, acts as an inhibitor of protein digesting enzymes, but amylase will deactivate hCG along with trypsin. (http://www.navi.net/~rsc/sialo.htm).

[103] Rolfe, R.D. (Mar-Apr., 1984) Interactions Among Microorganisms of the Indigenous Intestinal Flora and Their Influence on the Host. Review of Infectious Disease, Vol. 6, Supplement 1. International Symposium on Anaerobic Bacteria and Their Role in Disease. pp. S73-S79. University of Chicago Press. Retrieved from http://www.jstor.org/stable/4453304

[104] University Of Ulster (2005, March 28). Bacteria Can Help Lower Cancer Risk, University Of Ulster Expert Says. *ScienceDaily*. Retrieved March 14, 2010, from http://www.sciencedaily.com /releases/2005/03/050325145217.htm

---

[105] American Association for Cancer Research (2010, February 9). Soft drink consumption may markedly increase risk of pancreatic cancer. *ScienceDaily*. Retrieved from http://www.sciencedaily.com /releases/2010/02/100208091924.htm

[106] Goforth, E.L., Goforth, C.R. (2001) Appropriate Regulation of Antibiotics in Livestock Feed. Boston College. Retrieved from http://www.bc.edu/bc_org/avp/law/lwsch/journals/bcealr/28_1/02_FMS .htm

[107] Guide to Less Toxic Products (n.d.) Environmental Health Association of Nova Scotia Retrieved from http://www.lesstoxicguide.ca/index.asp?fetch=babycare

[108] Green, A. M.D. (2008, March 25) Navigating the Earache. Retrieved from http://well.blogs.nytimes.com/2008/03/25/navigating-the-earache/#more-177

[109] IBID

[110] Yogurt (n.d.) The George Mateljan Foundation Retrieved from http://www.whfoods.com/genpage.php?pfriendly=1&tname=foodspice &dbid=124

[111] Wollowski, I, Rechkemmer, G. and Pool-Zobel, B. (2001) Protective Role of probiotics and prebiotics in colon cancer. *Am J Clin Nutr*; 73 (suppl):451S-5S

[112] Guyenet, S.Ph.D.(2009, December 12) Butyric Acid: an Ancient Controller of Metabolism, Inflammation and Stress Resistance. Retrieved from http://wholehealthsource.blogspot.com/2009/12/butyric-acid-ancient-controller-of.html

[113] Practical Applications of Probiotics in Health and Disease (2008) Harvard Medical School, Division of Nutrition Webcast. Retrieved from http://www.presentme.com/harvard/oct2008.asp

[114] Probiotics Basics (n.d.) Retrieved from http://www.usprobiotics.org/basics.asp#role

[115] Kesslser, D. (13 March 2010) Obesity: The killer combination of sugar, fat and salt. Retrieved from http://www.guardian.co.uk/lifeandstyle/2010/mar/13/obesity-salt-fat-sugar-kessler/print

[116] Heber, D.MD, Bowerman, S. (2001) *What Color Is Your Diet?* New York: Harper Collins (pp.242-243).

[117] Frank B. Hu. (May 14, 2003) Overweight and Obesity Rates in Women: Health Risks and Consequences. Retrieved from http://www.medscape.com/viewarticle/452831

[118] Vigilante, K.,MD, Flynn, M (1999) *Low-Fat Lies, High-Fat Frauds and the healthiest diet in the world.* Washington, D.C.: Life Line Press, (pp. 41-42).

[119] Mayo Clinic (5 June 2009) Cholesterol: The top 5 foods to lower your numbers. Retrieved from http://www.mayoclinic.com/health/cholesterol/cl00002

[120] IBID – See citation 74.

[121] Batmanghelidj, F., MD (2003). *Water: For Health, for Healing, for life: Water & Salt, Your Healers From Within.* New York, Warner Books. (pp. 188-189)

[122] Black HS, Rhodes LE. (July 25, 2006) The potential of omega-3 fatty acids in the prevention of non-melanoma skin cancer. *Cancer Detect Prev.* 2006;30(3):224-32. Epub 2006 Jul 25. Retrieved from http://newsletter.vitalchoice.com/e_article000640081.cfm?x=b7TDVrT,b1kJpvRw

[123] Weatherby, C. (January 21, 2010) Omega-3s Slow Aging by Keeping DNA "Caps" Intact. Vital Choices Newsletter. Retrieved from http://www.imakenews.com/eletra/mod_print_view.cfm?this_id=1652450&u=vitalchoiceseafood&show_issue_date=F&issue_id=000418734&lid=bfGrWQm&uid=b7b1jv7h

[124] IBID

[125] IBID

[126] Miller, M., (n.d.) Breast Feeding and Mom's Diet Retrieve from http://www.007b.com/breastfeeding_intelligence_diet.php

---

127 Essential fatty acids and the brain. *Can J Psychiatry*. 2003 Apr;48(3):195-203.
"The ratio of membrane omega-3 to omega-6 PUFAs can be modulated by dietary intake. This ratio influences neurotransmission and prostaglandin formation, processes that are vital in the maintenance of normal brain function."

128 Sears, W. MD, (2009) *The N.D.D. Book: How Nutrition Deficit Disorder Affects Your Child's Learning, Behavior, and Health, and What You Can Do About It--Without Drugs*. New York: Little, Brown and Company, Hachette Book Group.

129 Long Chain Omega-3 Fatty Acids In Human Health: The Vital Roles of Eicosapentaenoic, Docasahexaenoic, and Alpha-Linolenic Acids (EPA, DHA, and ALA) (October 25, 2007) White Paper, Vital Choice. Retrieved from vitalchoice.com/uploads/WhitePaper.Omega3s.VitalChoice.NoCode.doc

130 Weatherby, C. (October 22, 2007), Omega Brain Theory Evolution Gets A Boost. Vital Choice Newsletter Archives. Retrieved from http://newsletter.vitalchoice.com/e_article000935502.cfm?x=b6P9VQK,b1pTrCB7,w

131 Fish and Omega-3 Fatty Acids (2010) The American Heart Association. Retrieved from http://www.americanheart.org/presenter.jhtml?identifier=4632

132 Omega 3 Fish Oil, Healthy Fats That Are Good For You (2010). Women's Health. Retrieved from http://www.womens-health-questions.com/omega-3.html

133 Sources and description for wild salmon. Retrieved http://www.vitalchoice.com/category/wild-salmon
134 Paiva-Martins, F. et al (2009) Effects of Olive Oil Polyphenols on Erthrocyte Oxidataive Damage. Molecular Nutrition & Food Research, University of Porto, Portugal.

135 Cicerale, S., Lucas, L. and Keast, R. (February 2, 2010) The Biological Activities of Phenolics in Virgin Olive Oil. *Intl. J. Mol. Sci.* Retrieved from http://www.gustrength.com/nutrition:olive-oil-phenolic-benefits

[136] Perricone, N., MD (2002) *The Perricone Prescription: A Physician's 28-Day Program for Total Body and Face Rejuvenation*. New York, Harper Collins. (pp. 67-70).

[137] IBID, 69
[138]Coconut in Medicine. The Healing Power of Organic Coconut Oil from the Philippines. Retrieved from http://www.cocofat.com/coconut-in-medicine.html

[139] The Water in You (n.d.). U.S. Geological Survey. Retrieved from http://ga.water.usgs.gov/edu/propertyyou.html

[140] Alcohol and Athletic Performance (n.d.). University of California San Diego Athletic Performance Nutrition Bulletinhttp://www.nmnathletics.com/attachments1/507.htm?DB_OEM_ID=5800
[141] Hydration, Why Is It Important? http://familydoctor.org/online/famdocen/home/healthy/food/general-nutrition/1013.html

[142] Maintaining Oral Hydration in Older People (2001) Best Practice. Evidence Based Practice Information Sheets for Health Professionals. Vol. 5, 1, Pg 4. Retrieved from www.joannabriggs.edu.au/pdf/BPISEng_5_1.pdf

[143] Hattersley, J. G. (2000). The Negative Health Effects of Chlorine. *The Journal of Orthomolecular Medicine Vol. 15, 2nd Quarter 2000.* Retrieved from http://www.orthomolecular.org/library/jom/2000/articles/2000-v15n02-p089.shtml

[144] Laino, C. Bottled Water Not Always Pure Water (2000) CNBC. Retrieved from http://www.drblank.com/hnbottle.htm

[145] Nutritional Care – Hydration (March2009) SCIEGuide 15: Dignity in Care. Social Care Institute for Health. Retrieved from http://www.scie.org.uk/publications/guides/guide15/mealtimes/hydration/index.asp

[146] IBID, 55 - See citation 117

[147] IBID, 27

[148] IBID, 122-123

---

[149] How much oxygen does a person consume in one day? (n.d.). Howstuffworks.com. Retrieved from http://health.howstuffworks.com/question98.htm/printable

[150] Torrey, T. (November 3, 2008) MRSA And Other Superbug Infections: From hospitals to the community, Superbugs Are Everywhere. About.com Guide. Patient Empowerment. Retrieved from http://patients.about.com/od/atthehospital/a/hais.htm

[151] IBID

[152] Ford, Debbie (2008). *Why Good People Do Bad Things: How to Stop Being Your Own Worst Enemy*. Harper Collins, New York. (p. 26)

[153] Anderson, Mike, (2009). The Rave Diet & Lifestyle: The Natural Foods Diet with Meals that Heal. www.RaveDiet.com ISBN 0-9726590-4-8 (p. 5)

[154] Anderson, Mike (2009). Eating- 3rd Edition. DVD (Amazon.com)

[155] Lipton, B.H. PhD (2009). *Biology of Belief, Unleashing the Power of Consciousness, Matter & Miracles*. Hay House, Inc. (pp. 101-104, 105-106)

[156] Feldman, R.S. (2010). Psychology and Your Life. McGraw-Hill, New York. Pp 336-338

[157] IBID, 103

[158] Amen, D.G. M.D. (2011). *The Amen Solution: The Secret to Being Thinner, Smarter, Happier*. Crown Publishing

[159] IBID, 1

[160] IBID, 1)

[161] IBID, 35 - See citation 155

[162] Fang, G., Hongtao, Y., Kirschner, M.W. (1998) Direct Binding of CDC20 Protein Family Members Activates the Anaphase-Promoting Complex in Mitosis and G 1. *Molecular Cell*, 2 (2), pp. 163-171.

[163]Bergman, J. (1999). ATP: The Perfect Energy Currency for the Cell. CRSQ Vol 36(1)

[164] IBID, 35 – See citation 4

[165] Lipton, B.H. (2009). *Biology of Belief, Unleashing the Power of Consciousness, Matter & Miracles.* Hay House, Inc
[166] Silverman, P.H. (2004). "Rethinking Genetic Determism: With only 30,000 genes, what is it that makes humans human?" *The Scientist* 32-33.

[167] IBID, 411-413 – See citation 148

[168] Stibich, M.,PhD (2009). Longevity: Why We Age – Theories and Effects of Aging. About.com Retrieved from http://longevity.about.com/od/longevity101/a/why_we_age.htm?p=1

[169] Pray, L.A. (2004). Epigenetics: Genome, Meet your Environment. *The Scientist* 14-20.

[170] Reik, W. and Walter, J. (2001). "Genomic Imprinting: Parental Influence on the Genome," *Nature Reviews Genetics* 2:21+

[171] Surani, M.A. (2001). "Reprogramming of genome function through epigenetic inheritance." *Nature* 414: 122-128.

[172] McCraty, R. and Tomasino, D. (2006) Emotional Stress, Positive Emotions, and Psychophysiological Coherence." Retrieved from http://www.heartmath.org/research/rp-emotional-stress-positive-emotions-and-psychophysiological-coherence.html

[173] McCraty, R., Ph.D., Atkinson, M., Tomasino, D., B.A., and Trevor, R., Ph.D *The Coherent Heart: Heart-Brain Interactions, Psychophysiological Coherence, and the Emergence of System-Wide Order.* Available through Heartmath.org.

[174] Pert, C.B. (1997). *Molecules of Emotion: The Science Behind Mind-Body Medicine.* New York: Scribner.

[175] Moyers, Bill (1992). *Healing And The Mind.* Doubleday, a division of Random House.

[176] IBID, 200

[177] IBID, 198-201

---

178 Frawley, David, PhD (1996). *Ayureveda and the Mind – the Healing of Consciousness.* Lotus Press, Twin Lakes, Wisconsin.

179 University of Arizona, Center for Integrative Medicine. http://integrativemedicine.arizona.edu/about/index.html

180 Science of The Heart: Exploring the Role of the Heart in Human Performance. Institute of HearthMath. Retrieved from http//www.heartmath.org/research/science-of-the-heart.html

181 Siegel, Bernie S., MD (1986; 1990 soft cover). *Love, Medicine and Miracles: Lessons Learned about Self-Healing from a Surgeon's Experience with Exceptional Patients.* Harper & Row, Publishers, Inc., New York.

182 Transcendental Meditation Clinical Research Published Journal Studies. Maharishi University of Management, Fairfield, Iowa. Retrieved from http://www.mum.edu/tm_research/welcome.html

183Sleep Drive and Your Body Clock (n.d.) National Sleep Foundation. Retrieved from http://www.sleepfoundation.org/article/sleep-topics/sleep-drive-and-your-body-clock

184 Besdine, R.W.MD (2007). The Aging Body. *Merck Manual.* http://www.merck.com/mmhe/sec26/ch320/ch320b.html

185 IBID (1)

186 The Franklin Institute (2010). The Human Brain. Retrieved from http://www.fi.edu/learn/brain/exercise.html#physicalexercise

187 IBID (1)

188 Wilber, D.Q. (Jan 31, 2007) FAA To Raise Retirement Age To Pilots. *The Washington Post.* Retrieved from http://www.washingtonpost.com/wp-dyn/content/article/2007/01/30/AR2007013001654.html

189 Buettner, D. (2009) Blue Zones. National Geographic.

190 Trends in Health Costs And Spending (2009) Kaiser Foundation. Retrieved from http://www.kff.org/insurance/upload/7692_02.pdf

[191] Klatz. R., Goldman, R. (2003) The New Anti-Aging Revolution. Stopping the Clock for a Young, Sexier, Happier You. New Jersey: Basic Health Publications. (p. 4)

[192] Wilson, J.F. (July 21, 2009). Can Disease Prevention Save Health Care Reform? *Annals of Internal Medicine.* Vol 151 No. 2. (p. 145)

[193] IBID (8)

[194] IBID

[195] IBID

[196] IBID

Notes — C VI:

[197] Klatz, R., MD, Goldman, R. MD (2003), The New Anti-Aging Revolution: Stopping the Clock for a Younger, Sexier, Happier You!, Basic Health Publications, Inc., New Jersey. Pp 4-5

[198] IBID, pg 13

[199] Boyd, Alan S. MD, Study on smoking and the skin published in the *Journal of the American Academy of Dermatology,* July 1999. Retrieved from http://www.east-westseminars.com/knowledge_base_research.php

[200] Oz, Mehemet C, MD, Roizen, Michael F, MD. *YOU: The Owner's Manual: An Insider's Guide to the Body That Will Make You Healthier and Younger.* Harper Resource (2005), First Collins Edition 2008

[201] Zani, Alexandra J. Skincare Product Selection Important to Medspas. *Dermatology Times* Aug. 2005. Modernmedicine.com

[202] Barrett-Hill, Florence, Advanced Skin Analysis, Virtual Beauty Corporation, Auckland, New Zealand, 2004. ISBN 0-476-00656-1

---

[203] Zani, Alexandra J. Advanced Skin Rejuvenation. *Beauty New Zealand*, July 2008.

[204] Zani, Alexandra J. Using New Technologies for Skin Therapies (laser & light therapies, microcurrent). *Beauty New Zealand*, November 2008.

[205] Goldberg, David J. MD,JD (2008). Laser Hair Removal, Second Edition. Informa Healthcare, United Kingdom www.informahealthcare.com

[206] NASA, LED-Based Lighting Treatment for Wound Healing. Retrieved from http://sbir.nasa.gov/SBIR/successes/ss/8-035text.html

[207] Whelen HT, Smits RL, Jr., et al (2001) Effect of NASA light-emitting diode irradiation on wound healing. J Clin Laser Med Surg. Dec: 19(6):305-14

[208] MediLabs, Wurzburg, Germany. Microcurrent and Body Sculpting with beautytek™ www.beautytek.org

[209] Microcurrents, Retrieved from www.midwestmicrocurrent.com/research.html

[210] Flanga V. Electrical stimulation increases the expression of fibroblast receptors for transforming growth factor-bets. *Jour Invest Derm*. 1987;88:488.6.

[211] Dayton PD, Palladino SJ. Electrical stimulation of cutaneous ulcerations: a literature review. Jour of Amer Podiatric Med Assoc. 1989;79:318-321.

[212] Botox Cosmetic® is a registered trademark of Allergan

www.ingramcontent.com/pod-product-compliance
Lightning Source LLC
Chambersburg PA
CBHW072144270326
41931CB00010B/1873

* 9 7 8 1 2 5 7 0 2 2 8 9 2 *